FOR THE BOYS

The War Story of a Combat Nurse in
Patton's Third Army

NCR DAVIS

For Tamara and Chris,
I thank you both for
your support.
Best Always,
Nancy 2023

CASEMATE

Philadelphia & Oxford

Published in the United States of America and Great Britain in 2023 by
CASEMATE PUBLISHERS
1950 Lawrence Road, Havertown, PA 19083, USA
and
The Old Music Hall, 106–108 Cowley Road, Oxford OX4 1JE, UK

Hardback Edition: ISBN 978-1-63624-158-6
Digital Edition: ISBN 978-1-63624-159-3

A CIP record for this book is available from the British Library

Printed and bound in the United Kingdom by CPI Group (UK) Ltd, Croydon, CR0 4YY

Typeset in India by Lapiz Digital Services, Chennai.

For a complete list of Casemate titles, please contact:

CASEMATE PUBLISHERS (US)
Telephone (610) 853-9131
Fax (610) 853-9146
Email: casemate@casematepublishers.com
www.casematepublishers.com

CASEMATE PUBLISHERS (UK)
Telephone (01865) 241249
Email: casemate-uk@casematepublishers.co.uk
www.casematepublishers.co.uk

For J, ever increasing

Contents

"So often they ask for their parents, especially, of course, for their mothers, and I've held many a boy's hand and pretended I was his mother at the end. I always say to them something like "better you should sleep. Everything will be okay when you wake up. Rest." And most of the time I've been lucky, and they close their eyes and die, thinking their mother's right there with them…"

Mary Balster, May 6, 1945

Acknowledgements

This story is based on material derived from the words of Lieutenant Mary Elizabeth Balster. While serving in the Army Nurse Corps (ANC) during World War II, the lieutenant wrote hundreds of letters to her St. Paul, Minnesota family. Inga Martinson Balster, her mother, had the foresight to keep the letters, hired a secretary to type them, and then had them bound chronologically, producing an archive of a young woman's first-hand chronicle of daily life in the ANC. The lieutenant also left a service diary and three photo albums. To support the archival evidence, I conducted interviews with Mary over a two-year period, from 2010 through 2012, and in the years following, I researched official army records and other historical texts. I also included content based on my own observations.

Had it not been for Sandra and Peter Riva, the archives would have remained lifeless. For many years I told myself that Americans were so enamored with the "15 minutes of fame" culture brought on by social media that there was no way that anyone would have interest in reading a story about an ordinary young woman who accidentally went to war a long time ago. But the Rivas argued that there would be interest in Mary Balster's story, that it did have value and should be told. As I look back on the many conversations we shared about writing and publishing, I realize that my insistence that no one would be interested in Mary's story served my subconscious need to keep a healthy emotional distance from the project.

Peter kept telling me to just write the truth, but I insisted that he should allow me to write the story any way that I wanted, which sometimes was all fiction, sometimes half-fiction and half-truth, sometimes three-fourths fiction and one-fourth truth. During this arduous process, he told me that some houses thought it had potential. But at the end of each conversation surrounding my latest iteration he'd go back to his original nudge, his notion that I should "just tell the truth."

But this is the truth about telling the truth: I didn't want to *tell* the truth because I didn't want to *face* the truth. Peter knew this, but it's not something that a person can tell someone else. What was he to do? Explain to me ahead of time that the only method for achieving the veracity the story deserved would be for me to go through an emotional abyss not unlike Demeter's search for Persephone? Peter knew that I had to become worthy of telling Mary's story and that the only way I could become worthy was to face a painful realization that Mary Balster, like millions of her peers, sacrificed her youth to a war that would ravage her innocent, beguiling, and magnificent spirit.

I hadn't wanted to face that realization because Mary wasn't just another war heroine who'd hired a writer to create a memoir of her time in the war. Mary was my mother. Nine years before her death, on her 90th birthday, she gave me her war letters and service diary. She told me that, as a nurse, she knew that she was losing her short-term memory. Before her long-term memory vanished, she wanted me to "edit" the archives. I wasn't sure what she meant by "edit," because my idea of editing wouldn't require her to tap into her long-term memory. Interviewing her, going through war photographs with her, researching her whereabouts in Normandy, homing in on the details of the injuries and illnesses of the soldiers who were her patients—these were not the stuff of editing. These were a full-time commitment to an overwhelming project that ended up consuming my life. "Editing" sounded reasonable. If she'd said that she wanted me to build a manuscript based on her war archives she knew that I would have replied with the truth—that I didn't have the time.

My life, like every other woman's life in her 40s, was complex. Taking on an editing job would sound a lot more palatable to me than what she probably knew that I was in for. So, Mary did what had been her habit since childhood. Manipulative as ever, she diminished the project by using the word "edit" so that I would take it on.

I flew back to Texas from Richmond with the big red volume of letters packed in a carry-on. The service diary was slim enough to fit in my purse, so once the plane reached altitude, I pulled it out and pondered the answer my mother had given me the day before I left.

We were standing at her bedroom dresser when she handed me the diary. Her hands seemed blue, caused by those pronounced veins that lined her thin skin, the indelible marks of a human being whose time on the planet has been longer than most. I flipped through the diary's yellowed pages and noticed that her last entry was May 5, 1945. I commented that there was a discrepancy. Her war letters' last entry was October 31, 1945.

What happened to the diary entries chronicling the last five months of her time in post-war Germany? Frayed threads served as evidence that the last section of the diary had been ripped out. On the plane, I smiled and shook my head when I thought back on her answer. It was so typical of her. She was evasive at best. She gazed down at her pink velvet house shoes and said, "Oh, you know, I was young and stupid. There's no telling why I did that!"

On that flight, I naively thought that the missing section of her service diary was of little consequence. After all, I couldn't very well "edit" pages that had been thrown away decades before I was born. My plan was to simply focus on the archives that she'd given me. In addition to the diary, I counted over 600 letters. Later, the next time I visited Mary, she handed me over 100 photographs of her time in the war.

It was once I began the task of reading those archives during the next few months after her 90th birthday that I realized this was no "editing" job. It would be up to me to unravel the sugar-coated letters that only served to provide strong hints that all was not right with love and Mary's war. The letters and the diary took on a new function. They were teasers. What was the real story of my mother's life from 1943 until 1946? It would take more than a decade for me to find a way to tell the truth of those years.

After each failed iteration, Peter and Sandy continued to have faith in the project and were confident in my skills as a writer. And they promised that I would eventually discover and develop a narrative voice that I had trapped and buried under a pile of counterfeit voices. After each misstep, I'd rant and bellow, sometimes for months, then coo like a bored baby in a crib for a while, and then crawl back to the laptop to begin again.

One day, after having spent a week with the Rivas, they told me that the process is slow for many writers and that the project might take me eight years. They were wrong. It took me 12. I remain in awe of the Rivas. They're uniquely devoted to representing authors who write about people like Mary who exemplified humanity at its best, especially during a time when much of it was at its worst.

NCR Davis

Author's Note

This book is based on my mother's recollections leading up to and including her participation as a combat nurse in the ETO, European Theater of Operations, 1943–1945. Students of history might be tempted to compare events mentioned herein to those gleaned from academically respected contributions that chronicle this same period. And certainly, while this work holds many historical underpinnings, I am not an historian. I'm a storyteller. In addition to the archives my mother gave me and the interviews I held with her, I grew up hearing innocuous anecdotes about some of the caregivers, especially Mona, Alabama, and Lorraine. Notwithstanding Lorraine, whom I met when I was 16, I never met the rest. But I felt as if I knew Mona, Alabama, and many others I've characterized because I'd heard the innocent stories about them during my formative years, decades before I ever had an inkling that one day my mother would ask me to honor them through a manuscript.

But the harrowing events, the gut-wrenching stories, weren't ever mentioned during my youth. My mother didn't share these private, painful recollections with me until almost 70 years after the war. Additionally, as her interviewer, I often witnessed her tendency to wear the proverbial rose-colored glasses when I pressed her for more specificity. It became obvious that she glossed over certain events, probably to shield herself from an emotional pain so fierce that she didn't want to touch it. I also picked up on certain body language that, to me, looked like fear. There were times when she wouldn't look at me, when her hands shook holding a spoon, when she pretended not to remember certain people.

At times, I got the sense that she was afraid that I was judging her, especially when I asked her about some of the choices she made during that time in her life. But the writer in me had to press her. I didn't want to. I loved my mother. It was horrible of me to ask so much of her, and I'm sure that I'll carry grief until my dying day for pushing her to revisit certain events.

As it is with most authors, the physical act of writing can reveal to us larger truths. Sometime during the writing of this work, I discovered a truth about choices; that is, when humans are participants in war, their present and future choices are greatly influenced because of the trauma they experienced.

For most of my life, I saw my mother make choices that I could not understand. But after writing several iterations of her story, I began to see that the trauma she endured during that time not only informed the choices she made back then but greatly affected choices she made for the rest of her life. This discovery was transformational for me because I began to understand my mother better, and I also gained a perspective that has alleviated a lot of my own angst.

At some point during the writing of my most recent iteration, it occurred to me that I should try to practice what many in tech fields refer to as the "steel man" approach, to go beneath the surface of others' choices, ponder why some make choices that seem abhorrent, stupid, self-serving, political, even cruel.

When I practice this approach, I've found that I'm more inclined to see what I have in common with those I've impetuously deemed as "lesser" because of their choices. The result is soul-satisfying. I've found that I live a freer life, one that tempers my insidious need to criticize and, instead, allows me to practice more humility and compassion. For all the gifts my dear mother bestowed upon me while we were on this planet together, this realization has been the most life changing, especially because I now believe that my mother was hoping that by choosing me to tell her war story, I would learn to have a more open attitude, a less critical nature. Until recently, I assumed that my mother chose me to write her war story because I was the only child of her six to hold degrees in Literature. Now I believe that my mother chose me to write her story because a mother knows her children. I think she chose me because she knew that I needed to go through the process more than her other children. I had the most to learn about life. She wanted to make sure I learned it and knew that going through this experience with her would grow me up.

And I think she wanted me to see that she was just like I was as a girl, one who had all the aspirations to become a Cinderella. Her descriptions of her girlhood helped me to understand that she held the same hopes tied to the Cinderella myth that I grew up with and, for that matter, a lot of girls dream about even now, in the 21st century. Maybe she wanted me to understand that her Cinderella myth was decimated by war and caused her to make choices that others, including me, might not ever understand. She wanted me to finally understand that, for her, because of the trauma she endured, they were the only viable choices she could make.

And maybe there was another reason she asked me to embark with her on this project. Maybe she thought if she finally told me her story, including the private experiences that she had never shared before, she could let go of that wicked albatross of trauma that hunted her, haunted her, hung about her neck all her days. Maybe she hoped that the albatross would finally leave and allow her a little peace in her last years. It did—but only when she left her withered frame for good at age 99. For the departure of that albatross from my beautiful mother, I am relieved. No, scratch that. I am overjoyed.

NCR Davis

Preface

December 18, 1944
Somewhere in France
Dear Mother and Daddy,

... Just came back from taking a shower and now am sitting by the oil stove drying my hair before I go to chow. Mona is still in bed, so I just got a pail of water, and I'm heating it for her. She hardly ever gets up in time to take a shower that's from 4–5 for nite nurses but boy I wouldn't miss it. Got up at 2 today and washed clothes and ironed my fatigues. They finally got the generator working so we have lights now—blinking lights I should say as they keep going off and on and it takes forever to iron anything.

Last night the rush started at 9 p.m. and we never sat down once after that except for chow. The wounds were terrible last nite and the poor boys scared and wet and cold. We were busy giving hypos and repairing dressings etc. and as we are the admitting ward the backlog is terrific. One little 19-year-old boy received a back wound so had to lie on his stomach and when I went to give him a hypo his nose was just dripping, and he couldn't use his hands because they were wrapped in gauze and strapped along his sides, so I got some dressings to use for hankies and just had him blow his nose until it was all clean. Remember how you used to say, "now, blow," Mom? Well, I felt just like a mother then. He said, "gee nurse, thanks a lot," and the tears were rolling down his cheeks...

When 24-year-old Lt. Mary Elizabeth Balster wrote these lines to her St. Paul, Minnesota family, she was unaware that the date she penned—December 18, 1944—marked the first day of what historians would later describe as the Battle of the Bulge. Holed up with her evacuation unit in the Heinrich Himmler Barracks in Morhange, France, over the next six weeks of patient care in the 39th Evacuation Hospital she would see staggering numbers of casualties. Mary's unit would be one of a handful of Third Army hospitals set up just behind the front lines whose purpose was to care for the sick, wounded, and dying. The battle would become second only to D-Day in terms of American troop volume and blood spilled in World War II's European Theater. On lighter admission days, the evac's medical staff slept four hours out of 24, but two for every 24 was more the norm. When there was time to talk, usually during a 10-minute break for chow, she, other nurses, physicians, corpsmen, and engineers of the 39th Evacuation Hospital would debate what day it was. None of them could remember.

PART I

St. Paul, Fort Leonard Wood, Middle Tennessee Winter 1933–Winter 1943

CHAPTER I

On a Streetcar, Guilt Takes a Prisoner

Like most of Bette Balster's apparel, the coat had been a gift from her father—double-breasted wool that fell just below the knees. He'd advised her to avoid wearing reds with yellow hues. They clashed with her violet-grey eyes, raven hair, and olive skin. The coat, then, a cherry-red with blue tones, proved exceptionally stunning. The pumps were choice, silver "Enna Jetticks" that added two inches to her 5'4" height. Altogether, she often commented that this ensemble, among many in her wardrobe, held the power to lift her mood.

Indeed, she felt "on the beam" at half past four on the afternoon of Sunday, December 7, 1941. The 21-year-old swaggered into the main dining room of the St. Paul Union Train Depot—her strides intentionally long, confident. She hoped her entrance might award her an approving nod from her father if he weren't too busy to catch sight of her.

H. C. Balster (Herman Carl) managed the food services within the St. Paul Union Train Depot; a bustling 24-hour dining hall, two soda counters, a coffee shop, and a new recreation center that housed a 12-lane bowling alley. Once Bette began pursuing her nursing degree at the University of Minnesota, Sunday afternoons evolved into the optimal time for catching up with "Daddy." Over chocolate malts the two typically droned over shared affinities—world politics, the latest "great read," and fashion.

Christmas was coming, so on this visit Bette planned to deflect any tendency toward serious subject matter her father might be planning. She was set on spending a couple of hours chatting about Christmas and whether her beau Clinton would be joining the family for Christmas Eve dinner. And she hoped to relegate a few minutes to mention that she'd been considering a rather large purchase at Schuneman's Department Store (a mink stole) but needed

"Daddy's" sound advice regarding such an investment.[1] She'd argue that living at home was allowing her an opportunity to save a lot of cash. It was her final year of college, but she was being paid a stipend while fulfilling her nursing practicum at Miller Hospital. She also wanted to remind him that her food expenses were next to none. When she wasn't eating at home she was eating with Clinton, or she was grabbing free snacks in the depot's coffee shop. If by some slim chance her father brought up any sound argument against the stole, she was prepared to defend her stance by pointing out that it was the *ideal* time to purchase something extravagant. After all, discretionary money might not be so plentiful once she and Clinton married. He'd only begun his career as an engineer. And Clinton was "such a saver," choosing to continue living at Mrs. Fuhrman's boarding house despite his recent promotion, but that decision was because Clinton shared her mother Inga's penchant for austerity. They were both Swedes, which meant, in Bette's opinion, that they were both so cheap that they forgot how to have fun. Surely her father would agree that this was the time to get that mink, as Clinton and Inga would never approve; in fact, Bette imagined the two of them rolling their eyes at each other at such a ridiculous notion, so "better they should" *not* know about the purchase until after it was said and done.[2]

Just as she was counting on her fingers the reasons for the mink versus the reasons against, she saw that, indeed, her father had noticed her entrance, but even at 20 feet away, his gaze didn't suggest the amiable mood that she was expecting. She got closer. His eyes were beady, and they were fixed on her. Then his eyebrows started moving so near each other that they became one bold line. In fact, at that moment, one might very well be reminded of Teddy Roosevelt's forehead on Mount Rushmore with those carved lines, cut so deep and serious.[3]

Even though the sound of her father's voice had been predicated by the scowl, it threw her into a bit of a jolt, particularly since it had been loud enough to cause a sharp echo. The utterance, only two syllables in length, "Ma-ry," embarrassed her since both of her parents addressed her by that God-given

---

1   Schuneman's and The Golden Rule, which locals referred to as "The Rule," were two iconic general goods stores in St. Paul during the golden age of department stores.
2   "Better they should," or "better I should," was slang popular in the 1940s, especially in the mid-west.
3   Mount Rushmore, the national park, had been officially opened to the public only a few months prior to the attack on Pearl Harbor.

name only when she was "in a little Dutch."[4] And that simultaneous pressing of his forefinger hard into his mustache—altogether it was just too much. If the gods had given her a choice between staying there and enduring the shame or melting into the floor, she would have chosen the latter.

Essentially, he'd "shushed" her in front of the patrons and his wait staff as if she were an unruly child misbehaving in church. It seemed that throwing him a searing stare was absolutely in order, but she decided against it. In the next couple of seconds, her intuition superseded her embarrassment. Something odd was going on in that dining room. Was her father's unexpectedly tense mood warranted?

On her father's command, one of his new hires, a young man who looked to be around 19, ran to the depot's newsstand counter and reached behind it to tune the radio and turn the volume knob to maximum. Mary slid into an empty booth and unwrapped a blue wool cowl from her neck. With a collective gaze at the loudspeaker, wait staff, patrons, and her father held a unifying disbelief, as if their collective reaction to the news might magically erase what they were hearing.

The Japanese had attacked Pearl Harbor.

She looked toward her father. His big brown eyes welled. He grimaced and stooped, as if he'd just suffered a physical blow to the gut. For the first time in her life, she saw hints of an old man. And in the few minutes that it took her to recognize the gravity of America's new incarnation, she was changed, too.

From that day forward she would be known as Mary. Remnants of Bette wanted to race toward her father to offer a daughter's hug, but Mary decided against it. He wouldn't want any consoling gestures that would suggest to onlookers a vulnerability, even though their entire world felt wrecked and lost. Bette would have run to her father. Mary didn't. Bette was the name they called her during girlhood. Mary would be the name of her adulthood and, indeed, in that train depot's dining hall, it felt like it was time for everyone in America to grow up.

She'd gone there to share a chocolate malt with him, but after the news of that afternoon, anything that might be considered even remotely extravagant seemed suddenly inappropriate. After a couple of hours that she mostly spent eavesdropping on her father's conversations with other men as they speculated on what would be next for America, she decided there was no use remaining at the depot. She was certain that the news would cause her insomnia. She

---

4   "In a little Dutch" was 1940s slang that meant a person had been reprimanded or chastised for inappropriate behavior.

should get home and prepare for bed as early as possible to allow at least three hours of the tosses and turns she knew would be coming. Despite the attack at Pearl Harbor and the likely outcome that her country would declare war soon, she would be expected to report for duty at Miller Hospital at seven the next morning.

When she bid him a good night, he touched her young face with his thumb to wipe the dribbles of mascara. His daughter's cheeks still boasted baby fat, round and full.

Just outside the depot's main entrance, she stopped on the sidewalk to feel for her long locks of black curls, tucked them under her red beret, then wrapped her neck in the wool cowl that her sister Nancy had knitted. She paced briskly to catch the streetcar. Snow dew melted on her eyelashes and tingled her nose and cheeks. She reached for a Kleenex to dab her face.

It was meant to be a white Christmas again, so the weather prognosticators had promised, and even though she'd lived in St. Paul her entire life, every new snowfall piqued Mary's sense of adventure. After all, it meant that she and Clinton could track fresh trails with their cross-country skis. And there would be a chance the lakes would offer them a longer ice-skating season. Unlike her mother, Mary loved the snow and had never thought of it as burdensome.

But that evening, as she stepped onto the streetcar and found a seat by a window, she peered out, saw the speckling flakes beneath the streetlights, and felt nothing. She recalled the conversation she'd overheard between her father and a long-time patron of the diner. They'd been whispering that some of the boys at Pearl Harbor were probably trapped in their submarines. She conjured hopeful images of ways they might survive, get free from the subs' bowels somehow.

But if they couldn't get out, would they suffocate? Or drown? To replace these horrifying images, she looked out the streetcar window to view sights of the town she loved. The snowfall hadn't changed. There was no wind, no storm, just snowfall, silent and heavy.

Weeping showed up, then all-out crying that she tried in vain to muffle with tissues. Soon she was reaching down deep into her right coat pocket to search for another clean tissue. It was empty. She'd have to rely on the drenched used tissues she'd stuffed in her left pocket.

The streetcar reached the stop closest to her parents' house. She walked the last couple of blocks toward "1262," the number of her family home on Stanford Street. She decided to try to figure out why the snow, at first, had no effect on her mood but in a matter of minutes it had moved her to sobbing. By the time she reached Stanford, she understood why. It was because the weather had not reacted to the news at all. The snow should have been ushered in by a howling and massive blizzard. The muted snowfall seemed like a sign from God that He didn't care about what happened to the boys in Hawaii. The serene snow that blanketed St. Paul was a white shroud of ambivalence. She wanted the night to fill itself with grief. She thought that everyone and everything, including the snow, should be outraged—for the boys.

At the depot, the speculation that night was that the United States would declare war. The next day that speculation was realized. Soon every patriotic American devised their own plans for helping the cause. Mary was no different.

Of course, for a young woman, it would take a little more personal conviction and a lot more creativity than if she'd been born male, but she wouldn't allow the fact of her gender to get in the way. Just how she'd contribute she wasn't sure. The boys were going to need nurses, and her nursing practicum would be finished at Miller in late spring.[5] Then there'd be her graduation during early summer of '42, and then, after gaining some nursing experience, say, 8 or 10 months' worth, then, if the war was still on, she'd help take care of them.

Suddenly, by crafting a tentative plan, she felt slightly better, her wretched emotional state comforted with thoughts of pledging her life to her country's service. And, truth be known, just a few weeks before the events of that afternoon, she'd already begun an evaluation of her place in the world. She'd already been pushing herself to make some changes, grow up a little bit. And after Pearl Harbor, the mink stole idea seemed to be another example of a long list of follies. Now she felt embarrassed to have spent so much time imagining her strolls about town in that mink. It was just a provocative but false announcement to the world that she'd entered adulthood. Wearing a mink didn't make her an adult, for God's sake.

After Pearl, suddenly she grew tired of being perceived as impetuous, immature, bratty, self-indulgent, but she only had herself to blame for this reputation. Notwithstanding her choice to become a registered nurse, she'd never planned and carried out any other major life decision.

But as time moved past the shock of Pearl and the onset of world war, Mary thought less and less about the outrage and more and more about the notion that joining the service would offer her the opportunity she'd been looking for—to care for the boys who had a chance to live, and elevate others' estimation of her worth. Caring for patients satisfied her soul. But to use her nursing skills to elevate her ego was also important to her. She couldn't lie

---

5   Miller Hospital was a private hospital that catered to St. Paul's wealthy.

to herself about that. Joining the war effort had a definitive romantic allure. Men could be heroes. Why not women?

In the spring of 1942, Mary graduated from nursing school and started full-time work as a registered nurse at Miller. After five months of employment, her desire to join the war effort had manifested into a plan to join the ANC (Army Nurse Corps), but trepidation crept in every time she thought about telling Clinton. She grappled incessantly with her decision, as she knew he'd fight her. He might cut off his affections, or worse, try to talk her into marrying him. And it wasn't as if she didn't want to marry Clinton, but she felt that getting married would get in the way of serving her country. That would certainly count as some sort of mortal sin, as service to country in the Balster family held equal weight to their Lutheran faith.

Predicting Clinton's reaction to her plans of joining the service caused anxiety, no doubt. That worry compounded each time she imagined how her parents would take the news, especially since their new refrain at the dinner table was to "thank God in heaven" that their three children were girls. Every night it seemed that her dad announced the news of another friend's son who had signed up.

Her agony over where and when to broach the subject to beau and family resolved itself before she'd hinted at her plan to any of them. First, the discussion with Clinton never materialized because he was called to Florida for basic training. And, within weeks of Clinton's departure, fliers were posted at Miller's nursing wards announcing that the young student nurses in training at the University of Minnesota would be "paired" with "experienced" nurses already employed at the hospital. Mary and her fellow registered nurses were to train the student nurses who would then be deployed rapidly to care for the boys overseas.

The announcement set Mary off a bit. She felt insulted that less experienced nurses were to do the job for the boys that she felt was hers to do. She'd been waiting to gain more nursing experience herself and yet Uncle Sam was willing to recruit nurses with even *less* experience. Exasperating, to say the least.

If she had not been quite as stubborn, Mary's need to commit to the war effort could have been satisfied solely by training the student nurses and caring for long-term patients who'd returned from fighting in the Pacific and North Africa. After all, most people would count her nursing during this time as an indirect means of doing her patriotic part.

But that didn't feel like enough. She had promised herself that she'd join for the boys and couldn't remember a time when she'd ever broken a promise to herself or to anyone else. If the workload didn't let up by the middle of

January, then she'd have to finagle an excuse to leave her shift just half an hour early some afternoon to catch the streetcar and make it to Fort Snelling in time to meet with recruiters.[6] She assumed that they didn't work past 5:00 p.m., so she'd need to leave Miller by 2:45. She penned an exclamation point on Friday, January 15, signifying that this was the day—absolutely the last day—to broach the subject with H. C. and Inga.

She convinced herself that the bold mark on her calendar would somehow magically stuff her with the courage to tell them and then, finally, her service life would be a reality. But after each long shift at Miller, Mary collapsed on her bed at 1262 Stanford and gazed at the January 15 exclamation point, entranced with images of her parents' potential reactions.

Inga would say something rather stoic, and then she would eventually get inured to the idea and chalk it up to Mary's "typical impulsivity." But her father? There was no need to expend any energy imagining his reaction. No guesswork necessary. He would throw a conniption.

He couldn't stop her. She was a registered nurse, for goodness' sake. She was a grown-up, for Christ's sake. She was joining, by God, and her father would just have to accept it.

But in the end, Mary took the passive route. She ignored the exclamation mark, allowed the sun to set on January 15, 1943, and promised herself that she'd come up with a new plan.

Like many of Mary's childhood friends, Lorraine Matzke had chosen nursing as a career. Though she worked at a different hospital, the two gals often met for breakfast at the depot's diner.

On a Sunday morning Lorraine mentioned that her hospital was participating in the service training program as well. That remark became the seed for Mary's new plan.

She'd get Lorraine to agree to sign up with her. She considered this to be such a crafty and brilliant idea because it would erase her parents' potential accusation that she had devised yet another ill-begotten scheme that would be added to the infamous list of Mary's antics. Certainly, her parents would be more apt to feeling at ease about her decision if she had Lorraine by her side. They loved Lorraine, and how many times had she overheard them comment that Lorraine provided a "steady influence" over her? How many times, despite her proclivity toward impulsiveness, had she been saved by Lorraine's cogent, rational personality… blah, blah, blah.

---

6   Fort Snelling was a recruiting station during both world wars and decommissioned after each. Various army regiments garrisoned the fort, beginning in the 1800s.

But by the time Mary had reached 18, she'd discovered that parents' assumptions about friends could be dead wrong. By then, she was a veteran at wearing the "good little girl" persona, especially to preclude unnecessary parental worrying. And Lorraine's devotion to Mary meant that most of the time she'd go along with her schemes.

So it came to pass that only a few days following breakfast with Lorraine, Mary pitched the army idea to her over a single cup of coffee and, voilà, she'd lassoed an army buddy. Their sign-up would have to wait, though, as the next four weeks vanished. In addition to their training duties, patient load was at an all-time high at each of their respective hospitals. Working overtime became the norm.

Finally, by late February, there was a reprieve from the workload. Mary boarded the streetcar downtown to take the 8-mile trip to Ft. Snelling. She'd meet Lorraine there. Just as she took her seat on the car, her peripheral vision picked up an image that felt familiar, prompting her to turn and look out the streetcar's window.

It was her father, his flowing, elegant gait materializing on St. Paul's sidewalks as if he were cross-country skiing. The best friend Mary ever had, dressed in one of his beautiful tweed suits, gliding and greeting each passerby with his genuine felicity, just going about his daily routine. And there was Mary—his eldest daughter—going about her daily business, too, except that hers was to sign up for the war effort behind his back. She felt sick.

Mary had spent her life seeking her father's approbation. She'd never lied to him. She'd never gone against any of his wishes. She wouldn't dare buy a dress or a coat or a pair of shoes without consulting him. But for the biggest decision of her life, she had chosen not to discuss it with him at all. She tried to swallow, but she couldn't salivate. Her heart raced; its thumping drummed in her dry throat. Guilt settled on her like a new skin.

She could not have known then that, for the remainder of her memory, she'd never be free of the guilt that became part of her that afternoon.

Loyal Lorraine was waiting for her by the rails. Once Mary was close enough for Lorraine to get a good look at her, it was clear something was wrong. Mary'd had a bad trip over, having seen her father on the street so "happy go lucky," ignorant of her plans. Lorraine felt like Mary's mother again, comforting her with maternal tones and reassuring hugs, but she hurried Mary along to get the task at hand completed, promising her they would talk more about it after they'd enlisted. On the streetcar back to downtown, Lorraine asked Mary why she'd chosen not to tell her parents, or at least why she'd not told her father, as everyone who knew the Balsters understood how close Mary and her father were.

He had served as a PFC, Private First Class, in World War I. Mary knew little about that time in his life, only that he'd often muttered to her and her sisters that they had "no earthly idea" how horrible it was. And how many times had they heard him scream during the night, her mother curtly explaining the next morning that it was nothing, that their father had just had a war nightmare. He would tell Mary no, absolutely not, end of discussion, and then Mary would feel conflicted, and then she'd feel guilty, and then she'd feel determined again. And it really would not make any difference because she had decided on December 7, 1941, that somehow, some way, she would join.

Lorraine assured her that nothing would be the same as it had been for her father in the first war. The fact that Mr. Balster had served in Normandy had nothing whatsoever to do with Mary signing up for the service. It would be completely different, especially the way that the Allies were ripping through North Africa. There was probably no chance at all that she and Mary would even get finished with training before the war would be over.

That evening Mary entered the front door of 1262 Stanford as a second lieutenant in the United States Army Nurse Corps. She'd been correct about her father. He threw a conniption.

CHAPTER 2

During Quarantine, a Nurse is Born

Nancy and Constance (Connie) Balster were inured to the impulsivities that characterized their older sister Mary and had often joked about their theory that she had been switched at birth. Every other member of the family, including Gram, their paternal grandmother, held to a life of organization and the utmost respect for rules. That Mary had joined the army seemed to be the height of irony to all the other Balsters. On the other hand, Mary typically made important decisions on a whim, so they figured that she had to have been overcome with the patriotism of the day. Fifteen-year-old Connie commented that at least Mary had possessed enough good sense to talk her friend Lorraine into joining the service with her.

Mary and Lorraine had met in the sixth grade, but their friendship was eternally sealed during their seventh-grade year when Mary contracted tuberculosis. It had been at the train depot restaurant that Mary and Lorraine witnessed the pale and worn faces of many patrons, guessing that they might be sick. By December 1933, the best friends had begun a regular attendance at funerals for parental friends memorialized at St. Paul's Cathedral, victims of tuberculosis.

Winter began its descent early that year, and its brutality held no sympathy for the many who had survived the Depression only to die from its cure. Work brought people together, their germs included. The WPA and other work programs had alleviated the economic ravages of the Great Depression, but a costly result was that infectious diseases such as TB spread, with more people in contact with others in the workplace.[1]

---

1   Tuberculosis has been called the most successful human pathogen of all time with a 35,000-year history. In the U.S., the 1930s outbreak had a direct correlation to the WPA (Work Progress Administration), the federal government's public works project that helped end the Depression but caused transient workers to spread infectious diseases like TB.

On a stark day, Mary noticed that the cathedral's domes held so much snow they reminded her of the dollops of whipped cream that decorated the chocolate malts she and Lorraine always ordered at the train depot's soda counter. She wondered how long it might take before she would feel like having a malt again. She didn't seem at all hungry of late, and her wool sweaters had begun to hang off her body so loosely that she could not keep warm.

The coughing started on Christmas Eve, 1933. Nancy played the piano while Connie led the family in the singing of carols. Both were talented in music, furthering their notion that Mary could not be related to them since she was hopelessly tone deaf. Perhaps because she had no musical ability, her adoration for music was heightened, much to the chagrin of the two sisters' ears, as she bellowed out notes too flat or too sharp. But on this night Mary coughed more than she sang, and Gram, a former nurse, became concerned.

Sometime after Christmas, Mary was admitted to the hospital. She was sputum positive for tuberculosis. During her youth, one in 170 Americans was sent to a tubercular sanatorium to either recover or die. These places of isolation were known as "death waiting rooms." As an avid newspaper reader, Mary was aware of them. So, when the doctor entered the hospital room to discuss her care with her parents and grandmother, she begged to remain home. Thirteen seemed too young an age to be sent away to die alone.

H. C.'s mother was a stereotypically industrious German who didn't know how to leisurely retire. One of her closest friends, a Mrs. Fuhrman, owned a boarding house, so when Gram retired from nursing, she began helping Mrs. Fuhrman with daily chores. Gram argued vehemently that her friend would support a leave of absence while she nursed Mary back to health. In fact, she would be relieved not to pay her, as currently the boarding house only had four tenants.

Gram was possibly fibbing about the number of boarders. Maybe Mary had inherited from her that willingness to pull guile out of her pocket if a situation called for it.

She was discharged from the hospital the next day and, by evening, H. C. had moved most of his mother's belongings from Ms. Fuhrman's to 1262 Stanford.

For the next 11 months, Mary was quarantined in her room, Gram at her bedside. During the first three months of her confinement Mary felt so weak that even uttering a whisper proved difficult. Her father bought a small chalkboard for her to write down any care requests. Before anyone had thought about it, she began writing her wishes in German, as Gram had been virtually the only person with whom she had contact. In addition, Mary felt most comforted when Gram read to her. And so it was in German that Mary heard her Gram's voice read *Little Women*, *The Secret Garden*, *Anne of Green Gables*, *Little Men* and *David Copperfield*. In her grandmother, she found her heroine and muse. By her 14th birthday Mary's health returned, and she announced to her family that one day she would become a nurse as a tribute to "Gram" for bringing her back to life.

But there were other less positive consequences associated with Mary's illness. A dysfunction arose in H. C. It was as if Mary's illness frightened him to such an extent that he unknowingly awarded Mary complete absolution for any future wrongdoing for the remainder of her adolescence. Nancy felt the sting of Herman Carl's sudden favoritism of Mary more so than Connie did, probably because Nancy was only two years younger than Mary while Connie was a distant six.

Nancy recalled a time not long after Mary's convalescence in which Mary decided to make chocolate eclairs that created a disaster in the kitchen and then had the audacity to leave it in that state. H. C. defended Mary's mess, stating something to the effect that Mary had "mastered quite a difficult recipe" and perhaps Nancy should clean up the kitchen to "help her older sister."

Such became the norm at 1262. Nancy compensated by choosing a life of extreme discipline, earning straight A-pluses, winning the state piano competition, learning to speak German with as much proficiency as Mary, all to win the respect and admiration of their father. And while he seemed very proud of Nancy's accomplishments, all paled in comparison to any activity Mary flitted about doing.

To her credit, Mary never held any critical thoughts toward those she loved. Those who knew the young Mary said that she had been born with an endearing compassion but being sick all those months and coming so close to death seemed to hone her empathic nature. She loved completely, ideally, loyally. And it was not as though Mary was unaware of her beneficiary status in all things Balster. If Nancy appeared jealous after their father had awarded Mary yet another undue courtesy, Mary would find some way to compensate. She invented ways to make Nancy feel better, usually by faking a need for her sister's help or manipulating facts and behaviors to make certain that Nancy was fairly compensated for her daughterly deeds, too. And if anyone was more astute than Mary, it was Nancy. She would go along with Mary's act and oblige her, "helping" any way that she could. And so, Nancy began to love Mary unconditionally, appreciating Mary's overt attempts at recompense for being their father's favorite.

Inga, always keen to Mary's craftiness, would sound the alarm if she suspected that Mary was "up to something," often following with, "You know your older sister is dumb like a fox." But neither parent was bothered by

Mary's amusements. Instead, they were humored by them. There was also that underlying reminder that they were so lucky that Mary survived TB. It would have seemed a bit like they were testing fate if they voiced any derogatory opinion regarding her antics.

During Mary's tuberculosis quarantine, Lorraine may have been the greatest sufferer. She wasn't allowed to visit for many months. To cope, Lorraine turned her solace in the direction of comfort food. By the time Mary was able to receive visitors, Lorraine had gained close to 30 pounds. In turn, Mary had lost 20.

Mary hoped that Lorraine's future growth spurts would alleviate the weight gain. But Lorraine seemed unable to force certain aspects of her body to mold into the proportions that Mary wished she could. It didn't help that Lorraine cared little about joining her for six hours of tennis and swimming each day during summer. Nor did she have any interest in skiing, ice skating, or sledding in the winters. Mary had no use for the inside, Lorraine no use for the out.

Because of Mary's active sports life, school popularity soared. Dates were too numerous to count. Lorraine fell to depending on Mary to land her some leftovers. So, Mary established a behavior of co-dependency concerning her relationship with Lorraine, just as she had with Nancy. To maintain equitable status among their friends, Mary behaved as though, if it were not for Lorraine, she could never keep up with her own head or body. In Algebra and Chemistry, Lorraine got credit for every great mark that Mary received, as Mary often claimed to Lorraine's mother, "Gee, Mrs. Matzke, if it weren't for Lorraine, I'd be failing!"

By the time Mary and Lorraine joined the service, most of their friends and family assumed that Lorraine was going to take care of Mary. No one, save for Nancy, Connie, and Inga, knew that Mary was quite capable of forging her own way.

Her clandestine trip to Ft. Snelling struck her father with a stinging set of emotions. War was in Europe. It was in the Pacific. And now his eldest had brought it to their home in a personal and terrifying way.

Virtually every American committed daily to the war effort at home. They gladly rationed staples like sugar and flour, planted victory gardens, participated in scrap metal drives, and purchased war bonds. In movies, in popular music, on billboards and propaganda posters depicting Rosie the Riveter and other cultural icons doing their part for Uncle Sam, the war saturated American culture.

For the life of him, he didn't understand why Mary couldn't be satisfied with the many opportunities for contributing to the war effort right in St. Paul. Instead, he was living with the unmitigated reality that of his three daughters, the one who'd come so close to death from TB only 10 years before had chosen to place her life in more peril than she could possibly fathom.

He worried incessantly about her personality—how it stood in direct contrast to all things army. It wasn't just her caprice that woke him during those nights. His mind wandered between his angst for having contributed to her sheltered upbringing and to having allowed her an arrogance that rules were meant for "ordinary numbskulls." Mary would not understand or appreciate the military. She was spoiled, obviously rebellious, never in agreement that rules were rules for a reason. Although Mary claimed that her parents had been as committed to their sense of patriotism as some Catholic families in their neighborhood were about their attending mass daily, he wasn't able to accept that his own sense of patriotism had contributed to Mary's decision. She insisted that it had, that the welling of emotion that she'd experienced on the afternoon and evening of the Japanese attack on her own country's soil was a natural consequence of a cultivated passion for patriotism.

But more than any other reason for his grief over Mary's decision was his own sense of regret for not having been more forthcoming about his own war experiences. He knew firsthand what she was headed for, and he couldn't help but wonder if his inability to talk to his family in any detail about his experiences in World War I had contributed to her naïve decision. If he'd had any inkling that she would ever contemplate serving her country by becoming a soldier, he would have been more open about World War I.

Finally, Mary helped him reach a resolve. Even if he'd been able to talk with her in detail about his war experiences, she wouldn't have been dissuaded. She'd inherited a stubbornness from both him and Inga.

The truth was that both he and Inga had suspected that Mary was planning something big. After all, she was their daughter. But they had assumed that it had something to do with Clinton. Many young couples were forfeiting the opportunity for grand nuptials and choosing elopement because of the war. And they saw Mary as one who wouldn't hesitate to do such a thing, given her tendency toward caprice.

Around the time that she began packing for her first assignment in the army, a letter from Clinton included plans for him to earn enough leave-time from Boca to spend a week with her at Fort Leonard Wood. But certainly, it wasn't a visit that would include elopement. Though neither Clinton nor Mary had said it aloud, there wasn't any real sense that either of them expected a long-term relationship would withstand the distance between them, much less the vast difference in daily life they now were facing. She packed his framed photograph but never consciously forced herself to consider whether the photo represented a future commitment, or if it simply served as just another St. Paul keepsake.

CHAPTER 3

Under Control

At 7:30 p.m. on March 31, 1943, Mary and Lorraine disembarked a government bus just inside the gates of their first post as second lieutenants in the United States Army Nurse Corps. Over Fort Leonard Wood, a spring moon reveled in pink and orange hues, but at less than a quarter in size, it proved insufficient for revealing any object beyond a flashlight's purview. As the bus pulled away and disappeared into the descending darkness, the batch of new recruits stood forming a haphazard line facing a young man saluting them. It was too dark to make out his rank but once everyone was within earshot, he introduced himself as a sergeant and said they were to follow him to the Officers' Recreation Hall. The commanding officer would be providing a welcome and briefing before the nurses would be taken to their assigned quarters. Someone wanted to know if they should try to find their belongings. The bus driver hadn't shown a great deal of care unloading them. They were strewn about so haphazardly that it would take an army to sort through what belonged to whom. But the sergeant ignored the question, so the recruits simply followed his wavering flashlight to the Rec Hall and figured someone else would take on that duty. The post felt so remote that if any of their belongings were to be rifled with while they attended the briefing, the primary suspect would most likely be a bear.

Although she remembered hardly any instructions given during the briefing, Mary recalled the chief nurse saying that she typically made all decisions regarding nursing assignments but that generally those decisions were based on the individual's civilian experience. If the nurse had more experience with medical patients as opposed to surgical, then more than likely that nurse would begin her stint at Ft. Wood in the "Medical Ward." In Mary's case, her only job post-graduation had been as a nurse on medical beds at Miller, so she reasoned that her first assignment would be on the Medical Ward and, conversely, that Lorraine's first assignment would probably be in surgery. Lorraine naturally gravitated to surgical nursing skills, having honed dexterous, nimble fingers from years of knitting, sewing, and crocheting.

After the briefing, the chief was extraordinarily kind to Mary. She let her borrow some evening dresses since there was a dance planned for the next night, having overheard Mary say that she hadn't packed any formal wear. The chief said she doubted that she'd need the dresses anyway because she'd received overseas orders. A new chief would be replacing her at Fort Wood by the end of the week.

Just after the briefing, scuttlebutt had it that her replacement, a Lt. Dorothy Maxson, had no interest in offering any such kindness toward the nurses who fell under her command, to which Lorraine whispered, "Well, isn't that just par for our luck? The nice one leaving. The mean one as replacement."

This "mean one" had been unable to greet the new recruits because she was working a night shift at the post's hospital, as nurse staffing had been cut short since most of the nurses had been transferred over recent weeks.

After some housekeeping announcements, a PFC and a military policeman (MP) escorted the newest recruits to a Red Cross car. In addition to Mary and Lorraine, three other nurses climbed into the back of their car, legs perched atop others', bunched and squeezed together like too many children on a hayride. One of the gals thought to ask about their belongings. The PFC said that they had been taken already to their quarters while they'd been attending the briefing.

The gals bounced about as the car bumped and dipped on a narrow and wet dirt road. When a jeep or ambulance approached, the driver pulled the car as far to one side as possible to allow the other vehicle to pass by. The five passengers were so exhausted that not even Mary felt awkward remaining quiet, although prior to getting in the Red Cross car Lorraine had told her that her ears were worn out with Mary's constant chatter to everyone and that if Mary had come across a bear, she would have introduced herself to him, too.

Mary was the fourth to be dropped off. Lorraine scowled and moaned, deeply disappointed that they were apparently not going to be housed in the same quarters. But neither of them had enough energy left to grieve that fact for too long. Secretly Mary was not unhappy about finally having a little time to unwind alone. Lorraine could relax anywhere anytime, but Mary, always the entertainer, needed forced time alone to accomplish R&R.

Her room was the last one on the hallway, a lucky proximity for a personality such as Mary's for nights like this one when she was so tired there was no possibility for engaging with another soul on the earth. After a quick perusal of her surroundings, she tip-toed down the hall to the dormitory-style community bathroom.

It was there that she met her first hall mate briefly, a gal named Mona, who had the biggest darn dimples she'd ever seen. And she was too kind, understood how tired Mary probably was, promised that they'd get to know each other soon. She left Mary to perform her nightly ritual—showering and rolling her wet hair.

At 22 years old, Mary had been living under an assumption her entire life that rolling one's hair on a nightly basis would lead to holy matrimony and eternal bliss. She had a voluminous amount of wavy hair that probably would have cooperated no matter how little she tended to it. But she was convinced that the painstaking hour it took to cover her head in "kid curlers" and sleep in them were sacrifices well worth the next day's outcome—the hairdo of the day, the "Victory Roll," popularly worn by Hollywood bombshells like Rita Hayworth, Betty Grable, and Veronica Lake. Originally, the army had created the "victory roll" term to describe the celebratory roll formation of an American fighter plane after having shot down an enemy aircraft. Chalk it up to propaganda or fashion's attempt to join the war effort, in Mary's mind the victory roll was practically a requirement for any American female wishing to get noticed.

Once she returned to her own room, she noted that the floor lamp would have to suffice as a bedtime reading light since there wasn't a lamp on the nightstand. But there wouldn't be any reading tonight. She needed to attempt sleep, so she clicked off the overhead light and made her way into the single bed housed in Nurses Quarters 106, Room 24.

With eyes closed, she began to watch a series of disjointed images in her mind's eye—the orchids in the St. Louis gardens, the dark path that led to her quarters from the dirt road where the MP had parked the Red Cross car, that gal in the bathroom, Mona, with dimples that looked like two deep crevasses on an otherwise perfectly round and ripe peach. But then there was that awful recognition—she was so overtired there was no way that sleep was going to show up. If she wrote a letter or two, maybe she'd be able to relax after.

She got up and turned on the floor lamp, reached for stationery and a pen on the nightstand, and used her Bible as a writing surface.

March 31, 1943

Dearest Family,

It's 10:30 P.M., my 1st nite in the army, and everything's under control. Arrived here about 7:30 and by now have unpacked, put things in order, taken a shower and put up my hair, and have done lots of talking. Everyone's extremely pleasant and we received a very warm welcome including that from the weather—not hot by any means—just nice.

Am glad we took the opportunity to take a look at St. Louis. Gosh knows when we'll see it again—from all reports, leaves are not too frequent and transportation facilities are not too good outside the camp. There's a Red Cross car that carts the nurses around the camp that seems much larger than I had anticipated, the camp I mean. Was telling you about St. Louis. Am very excited and confused so please forgive if this letter is not very well connected. Will do better when I calm down.

Saw those gardens Miss Camelia spoke of. Took a bus and a streetcar to get there, but it was worthwhile. They are beautiful—that new spring green is just beginning to appear here. Saw some real orchids too. Then back by bus to downtown St. Louis where we ate lunch at the "Forum" and back to the depot in time to catch the 2:15 train. My first impression of St. Louis was super and will be looking forward to the time when I can get down there again and I do mean down. Left Newburg about 6 P.M. and drove up here in a gov't bus. The ride reminded me so much of the drive up to Mt. Rainier. Not as scenic perhaps, but it was <u>uphill.</u> We never stopped going up until we reached this place that is really isolated. Nothing but hills for miles around. The closest town is Newburg, which is about 30 miles down, and the red cross car brought us to our quarters which are rustic but very well equipped. There are 5 nurses' houses with about 20 rooms in each house. Lorraine is two houses up. Rooms are single. Mine is a corner one so it has two windows. This is it:

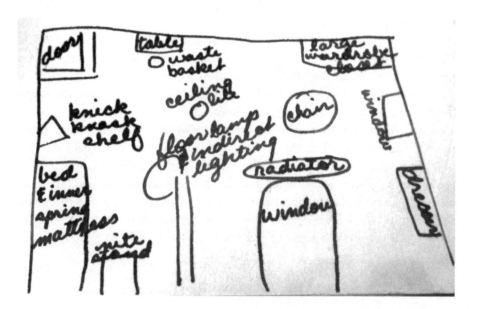

The furniture is all of dark brown metal and very nice. The walls and ceiling are like the inside of a cabin, but I'm very well pleased with the whole set up. There's a lounge, telephone, showers, bath, wash tubs, ironing boards etc. in each house. The rest of my environment is still a mystery and looks very complicated.

And, mother, do you remember saying that you thought you'd be sending something every week. How right you were. How would you like a small list right now.

1. 2 sheets and a pillow slip. (The army no longer furnishes them, and they are difficult to obtain here.) Throw in another washcloth and towel too if you can.
2. My cotton formal—there is a formal dance here every week and the girls say it's a "must have".

There are no bedspreads, curtains, dresser scarfs, but those can wait until I know more what the score is. We may not receive our uniforms for a couple of months as everything is so slow about getting here. If you could take care of those 1st items, tho, sure will make me happy.

Will meet the head nurse at 8 A.M. tomorrow, and I hope she's not as bad as her reputation—it's terrific.[1]

Well, seeing as how I have other corresponding to do (guess to who), better I should save the rest for later. Have not had a chance to get homesick, but just give me a few days. Everyone was so wonderful to me before I left, and I hope they know how much I appreciated everything. Please don't worry about me, the army has done a good job of taking care of us so far, but please write very often because I can see already how much those letters from home mean to everyone, and I'll try to do my best.

My address:
2nd Lt. Mary E. Balster, A.N.C.
Station Hospital
Fort Leonard Wood, Missouri[2]

(Will be waiting anxiously to hear from you.)

Greet the kids for me—especially Judy—tell them I will write tomorrow if I can.[3]
All my love to you all.
Mary

---

1   "It's terrific" had an ironic meaning. In 1940s slang, "she" or "he" is "terrific" meant that the referenced person's reputation was terrible.

2   The army broke ground on Fort Leonard Wood in December 1940. In the middle of the Ozarks, where winter and spring always bring inclement weather, thousands of workers were hampered but not deterred and, amazingly, construction was completed on 1600 new buildings. The army named the site after Major General Leonard Wood, a Rough Rider and surgeon from Spanish American War days whose second in command was Theodore Roosevelt. By 1941, field artillery battalions and quartermaster companies were also training there, and the installation also began serving as an engineer training facility. The growing need for engineers had outgrown facilities at other installations in the east such as Fort Belvoir in Virginia. Among the 1600 buildings constructed in only six months was a cantonment-type hospital, accommodating both surgical and medical patients. Despite the number of structures, Mary described in a letter that the post was, "really isolated … Recreational facilities are good … Six theaters, several officers' post exchanges, clubs, etc." https://home.army.mil/wood/index.php/about/history

3   Mary contended that Judy was her best friend "of all time," but since they did not share the same war experience Judy is not mentioned often in the war letters.

She noted the time and held off writing Clinton. Better to attempt sleep again. She'd grab a few minutes the next day to write him, or, better yet, she'd call him in Boca to let him know that she and Lorraine had arrived at their first post safely.

Earlier, her two windows' shades continually failed to stay down so she'd given up fighting them. Once she'd turned off the floor lamp this time, though, she realized that the broken shades wouldn't be a bother, as the small, persistent pink moon generated the only light coming from outside, producing soothing shadows, shaping the room's objects into a counterpane of soft angles. She moved about in the small bed twirling her arms and fingers to create her own shadows, intersecting hers with those produced by the nightstand, the floor lamp, the wardrobe, objects in her new life that seemed foreign and yet familiar. As she nestled into the single bed with the inner spring mattress, she felt oddly secure, which was initially difficult for her to understand when she considered that not only was this a strange new place to spend the night, but it was also a strange new life to spend from now on. To give herself some answer as to why this feeling of comfort had come upon her, she lay still and began to mull over the facts of her new incarnation. Nurses from civilian life who joined the army were given an officer's rank as second lieutenant, quite a notable distinction for any female who had no previous military training. She and Lorraine had not attended Officers' Training School, but like their male counterparts, females who held a degree were awarded an officer's rank by default, irrespective of any formal military training. The rank held a status she enjoyed thinking about.

When she'd disembarked the government bus and had been ushered to the briefing by that stoic sergeant, she'd doubted her own sense of authority, but the chief's welcoming words boosted her confidence that she held at least a fair amount. She was an officer, a rank in and of itself that awarded her an immediate sense of place and honor in a world dominated by men.

As she settled into a fetal position, it occurred to her that she, Lorraine, and the other nurses at the post outranked at least half the men there, maybe more than half. With this realization, sleep finally came, the quality of it better than it had been in some time.

The next morning proved far too busy for her to write Clinton more than a post card's worth of lines. Once that task was accomplished, she spent the remaining time allotted to jot a quick letter to family.

April 1, 1943

Dearest Mom and Dad,

Just a few lines before I prepare myself for the afternoon ordeal that starts at 1 p.m. It is now 12:15. Guess we are to get shots and a physical check-up this p.m.

Our morning consisted of signing our lives away. Must have written my name at least 100 times, fingerprinted again, interviewed by a staff sergeant who got me to giggling and screwed up all the information I handed out. We were then measured for uniforms and then to dinner. My mess ticket set me back $8.00 and is good for 24 meals. From now on I will eat only two meals a day. This noon was our first meal in camp—beans, brown bread, milk, cocoa, bacon, salad, and cake. Not too tasty but guess I'm not very hungry.

Expect to go on duty tomorrow that consists mostly of supervising and shoving a pencil from what I hear.

By the way, Daddy, when you start receiving war bonds and life insurance policies, keep them well-guarded for me, won't you? First, they told us we should buy a $25 bond each month and then they asked us if it was "OK." I have you and Mom signed up as my beneficiaries for my life insurance. We are required to have $10,000.00 worth. For a third person, I put Nancy's name. It will only be $5.00 per month and can be changed to a twenty-year endowment policy upon release from the army.

Also signed pay vouchers this morning. We get our checks April 30th. Receive reimbursement for our transportation before that, however.

There are five new nurses, and I'm the youngest. In fact, I am the baby of this house. Ages range from about 23–40. Green is no word for the way I feel.

Tonight, there is a dinner dance at the new recreation hall for officers and nurses. We barely got settled when someone had Lorraine and me fixed up with dates with some new lieutenants who arrived yesterday. It is formal, but they said it's OK to go otherwise as long as we're new. Am not too enthused about the idea as I'm still so confused but didn't want to be considered a "back-number" either. With all these men around don't see why Clinton couldn't be one of them.

I almost forgot—would you please send my tennis racket and a couple of balls? There are some very nice courts that I intend to take advantage of as soon as possible. Plenty of cakes, candy, etc., around, also billiard tables and ping pong in the mess hall—overall, quite a nice place.

By the way, tell Gram how good the cookies were. Had them for dinner last night and for breakfast this a.m., as we didn't get around to receiving our mess tickets 'til this noon.

Was glad for my new army blankets last night, as it got quite chilly.

Well, time is getting short and, as it takes us half an hour to find our destination, better I should start hopping. Will keep you well posted on my activities and hope for a letter from you very soon.

Mary

P. S. Let Nancy and Connie read these first impressions of an army nurse's life, won't you, and I will write to them as soon as possible.

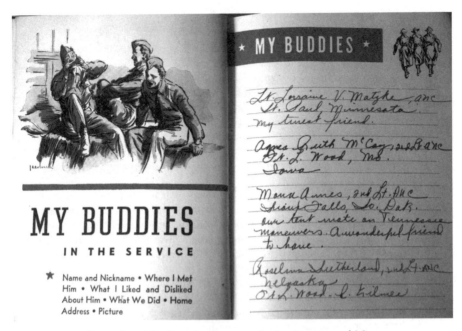

A page from Mary's service diary, mentioning Lorraine and Mona

CHAPTER 4

Mail Call

At 7:30 one May morning, Lt. Monica Ames returned to her quarters just in time to hold open its entry door for a private. It led them to the Common Room of Nurses Quarters 106. The PFC's hands toppled with a neatly stacked pyramid of boxes, seemingly all of them addressed to a Lt. Mary E. Balster. After confirming with Lt. Ames that, indeed, Lt. Balster lived in the building, he jaunted off to retrieve another stack from the jeep.

Mona cleared a few odd chairs from the back corner of the room to leave an open space for the bounty of letters, small packages, and large boxes that were postmarked as far back as, what, eight weeks ago. Yes, she'd let Lt. Balster know the mail was waiting for her, so the private bid her a good day. Then she ran after him, caught him as he climbed in the jeep. Was mail delivery to nurses' quarters a new perk? He didn't understand. She clarified. Would nurses still be required to stop by the mail room, or, from now on, would someone be bringing the mail to them?

That was a negative, the private said. Nurses would still need to go by the mail room. It was just that Lt. Balster didn't ever come by, and they didn't have enough room to store all her mail anymore.

The fact that all the mail belonged to Mary didn't really surprise Mona, but, in the two months she'd known her, she'd never caught Mary in a lie. In fact, she'd found her to be refreshingly genuine, so why in the world would she fib about going by the mail room daily and then proceed to seem so upset that her family still hadn't sent her a thing? She literally went around quarters whining that obviously she'd become her family's "forgotten lieutenant."

She walked slowly down the hallway, reached the last room on the left, and knocked softly. Then she let herself in, unsure if Mary was still sleeping. Even though she'd been on night duty, she guessed that Mary had probably been late returning to quarters after having been on another date with Zim.

But Mary was awake, sitting at her dressing table, donning her kid curlers and holding a tight grin. Her eyes shifted to the left and up to see Mona in the mirror's reflection.

"Hi," she said, with a hint of guilt in her tone.

Mona stood with her arms folded and asked her if she'd been doing something a little rebellious and to not dare fib to her.

Mary gestured for Mona to have a seat on her bed while she finished getting ready for chow. She was starving, as last night with Zim had zapped her of energy.

Mona watched this gal she'd known for almost nine weeks and already she felt an allegiance to her. It was as if they'd spent all their formative years together. Mary was so warm and generous. She shared her things and her thoughts so freely with Mona, so much so that Mona had told her recently that, while she was trustworthy, she was hoping that Mary wasn't so open with others who may not be that interested in her welfare. But Mary hadn't really understood that comment. She gave Mona that naïve, almost incredulous look, as if in disbelief that there was anyone on earth who would not have someone else's best interest at heart.

Mary's personality reminded Mona of a younger version of Norma Shearer when she played the wife of the unfaithful husband from that wonderful movie, *The Women*. Secretly, she hoped that Mary wouldn't have to endure the heartache and betrayal that Shearer's character went through before she learned not to award everyone the romantic assumption that they were inherently good.

As Mary carried on about her night with Zim, Mona took a seat on the bed. She gazed on with admiration. She loved Mary too much to envy her, but she often found herself wishing that she could have just a little dose of Mary's allure. The patients on Medical Ward had dubbed her "the pinup gal of the 39th." No wonder. She sat there with her straight posture and her full lips, chattering like a happy lark in sunlight. That sweet nature. That buxom figure. That silky black hair and those round cheeks that blushed without the help of makeup. A natural beauty with accidental charm. No wonder men adored her.

And there was Clinton's photograph holding its spot on her nightstand. But on the dressing table, a silver frame held a newer picture, one of her and Zim, along with Lorraine and her beau Francis, although everybody at the post called him Fran. Someone, maybe the post's photographer, had taken their picture at an informal dance. Fran was lighting a Camel for Lorraine. Since they were caught unawares, the photo captured such a becoming likeness of Lorraine. She was one of those who stiffened when she knew her photograph was being taken.

Mona left her perch on the bed, moved to Mary's side, and picked up the photo for a closer look. There, in direct contrast to Lorraine and Fran, were Zim and Mary, staring right into the lens and smiling confidently. They looked like movie stars. Mary was reticent to admit liking the image of herself, but it was her favorite picture of her and Zim together. It had been such a fun night for them. Mona teased her. As late as she was last night, it must have been even more fun.

The four had been inseparable ever since Mary and Lorraine's second night at Fort Leonard Wood. And it wasn't a matter of convenience for the two to exclusively date Zimmerman and Francis. Simply put, the four got along "swell." They attended any activity offered to officers on the post, from movie nights to informal dances. At the formals, cover bands played all of swing music's finest—Artie Shaw, Glenn Miller, Count Basie. So, unless Mary or Lorraine was assigned night duty, they never skipped out on the chance to engage in any rec time. Often, after a dance or a movie, the four could be seen traipsing over to the Officers' Club for late-night dining on deli sandwiches, popcorn, and cokes.

Mona helped her unleash the locks of velvety hair from the kid curlers as Mary was saying that the last two months were most assuredly the happiest time of her life, and she was almost certain that she would marry Zim. She'd fallen for him fast and hard. Mona was happy that Mary had found love. She hated to bring up the obvious, but she sure hoped that the war wouldn't get in the way of their plans. They probably should hurry up and get married, though, preferably before Clinton showed up or Zim got deployed. Or had she taken care of the Clinton problem?

Of course, she hadn't had a minute to even think about how to break things off with Clinton. And the latest news from him was that he would be taking leave from Boca to visit her in the next couple of weeks. She needed to call him, stop him from coming, just explain to him that she'd met someone else. Just tell him outright. But she just couldn't. She could if only he hadn't been admitted to the Medical Ward in Boca for a persistent eye infection. She just had to let his eye heal before telling him that their engagement was off.

As she anxiously droned on about her Clinton problem, Mona knew there was no use asking exactly how his infected eye had any relevance or correlation to breaking up with him. It wasn't as if he were dying, for Christ's sake.

***

Since Mona had just returned from night duty and Mary was now preparing to report for night duty on the same ward, Mona voiced her concerns about two patients, one who might be suffering from a grave heart condition and another who had contracted a nasty pneumonia.

Mona said that the heart patient was to be transferred, possibly to Minnesota, for further diagnostics, if they could get him stable enough. Both were certain that boy would never see combat and would be lucky to see 21. As for the pneumonia patient, there was some improvement, but Mona said to watch his fever. It had spiked last night. Mary said she'd watch him carefully.

Mona thought it a bit ironic that she knew Mary would do just that. Her care for patients was impeccable. But the question at hand was why Mary took little notice or care for the details regarding her personal life.

"Why? Oh, you mean because you found my dog tag in the shower?"

Mona chuckled. She was more intrigued about why there were upwards of ten, maybe 12 packages and four huge boxes and probably 20 letters from Minnesota piled in the Common Room. The only thing missing was a Christmas tree but, since it was May, she guessed a Christmas tree would look a bit odd.

Mary shrieked.

Together they ran down the hallway and, at the sight of the mother lode, Mary stopped. She grabbed Mona's arm, saying, "Oh my God, they didn't forget me. Oh, Mona. What in the world? Where? How?"

Mona said she didn't have a clue, that she'd let in a private who said they no longer had room for all of Lt. Balster's mail in the mail room. She had to ask. Did Mary fib about going to the mail room every day? Of course, she hadn't fibbed, and then she picked up the top letter. The mailbox number that Inga had written was the reverse of the box's number that Mary had been asking the mail room attendants to look in. No wonder there had been a mix-up.

Mona helped Mary carry the parcels back to her room. There was no time to open any of them now. Mary had to get ready for duty.

Mystery solved. Her family loved her. And Mona was relieved to know that Mary's character remained pristine.

Mona was getting tired but wanted to ask Mary's opinion about that patient who'd said his hearing was awful, the one who was afraid that he was going deaf. What was Mary's read on him?

Methodically, Mary pulled her russet shoes from underneath the bed. On top of it, she laid out her starchily pressed day beige uniform. Then she smoothed out her stockings.

Also under the bed, she'd stored her newly arrived overseas cap and sweater and two pairs each of GI white and GI black shoes.

Once their dress blues arrived, could Mona remind her that the day beige uniforms weren't allowed to be worn after 5:00 p.m. She was sure to forget that. The army had way too many stupid rules.

Then, logically, she laid out her read on the patient. First, he hadn't mentioned anything about hearing loss upon admission. His chief complaint at that time was that he was experiencing rapid heartrate and palpitations that he said had occurred repeatedly on maneuvers. But, what, he'd been on Medical for a week of observation, and there were no findings of palpitations, pain, dyspnea, or edema. And he hadn't suffered from rheumatic fever as a child.[1]

And did Mona know that the ward officer had told him that with no heart findings he would be discharged to return to maneuvers and that the palpitations he'd experienced on maneuvers were possibly related to heat intolerance? He was assured that his body would acclimatize. So now, suddenly, the guy claimed that his hearing was also a big concern and he wondered if his lack of hearing may have caused him a nervous condition that resulted in his heart palpitations. So, God should strike her dead if she was wrong, but it was her strong opinion that he was simply a very poor soldier and had gotten wind of certain physical conditions like heart defects or deafness that would guarantee him an honorable discharge. With full benefits, mind you.

She added that there was a circular from the Surgeon General's Office. She'd put it in the nurse's notes for Mona to read on her next shift. Mary had read it a few nights before. It highlighted a method for determining real hearing loss from fake. She was certain after reading the circular that the patient was just one of those rare birds who didn't belong in the service because he would make one excuse after another until he found some way to be discharged. She had no respect for him whatsoever and told Mona to stop feeling guilty about missing something. He was behaviorally disabled, not physically in any way, shape, or form. Just a trickster from the word go.

Mona read the circular the following morning, directed the hearing test, and, indeed, found there was nothing at all wrong with his hearing.

***

Mona and Mary looked forward to the following Saturday, as neither was on the shift schedule. Their only mandate was to attend the film *The Nazis Strike*

---

1 Dyspnea means shortness of breath; edema means swelling. Rheumatic fever as a child can cause permanent heart damage. The patient had not reported ever having had rheumatic fever, so there was even less likelihood that his claim of heart trouble was valid.

Malingerers were rare but occasionally the nurses came across them. They referred to them as "very poor soldiers," and felt that they should be allowed to leave the service since they probably were not going to be reliable in the face of battle.

A few patients were diagnosed with TB in April, but most on the Medical Ward at Fort Leonard Wood were either cardiac, ulcer, or hernia patients. Some patients were designated as "convalescent," which meant that they could be in the hospital up to 180 days. Mary mentions them in a letter to Nancy: "The convalescent patients do dishes on our ward and help me serve the food to the sick ones (mostly cardiac and ulcers)."

that morning.[2] Mary planned for their afternoon to include a grand opening of the mother lode of mail. She would ask Zim to pick her and Mona up that afternoon. He could borrow a jeep and pile the boxes in the back. Then they'd drive to the top of one of Fort Leonard Wood's highest hills, picnic, and open the boxes to share in the bounty. But what if the weather stunk, like it had for weeks? It might still be awful rain on Saturday, but one could hope.

There'd been so much rain that lone boots stuck in Missouri mud could be seen all over the landscape. Zim said that if you could see those abandoned hiking boots from an airplane, they'd look like small tree trunks, so random and odd. They were indelibly an absurd testament to the amounts of rain that had befallen the Ozarks that spring.

Saturday proved no different. The rain was tireless. When they returned to quarters after watching *The Nazis Strike*, Mary called Zim. She was distressed that the picnic plans were ruined. But it wasn't a problem. Zim would meet the gals in the Common Room. He'd be there by 3:00 p.m. Over the phone he reminded her that there was another formal that night, lest she forgot.

She hadn't and was hoping that one of the boxes from home would contain a few formals that she'd requested Inga to send for her and Mona. From now on, Inga should assume that she had twins in the service because Mona didn't come from a family of means and was a true peach of a gal, mid-western in every way, an absolute saint and best friend. Inga should send two of everything, from lipstick to perfume, hosiery to shampoo.

She often prayed that wherever Good Ol' Uncle Sam decided to send her, he'd send Mona there, too. That would make anything okay, although she sure hoped that Lorraine was right that the war would be over soon and that they could serve the army at Fort Leonard Wood for the duration.

Zim, as thoughtful a gentleman as one could ever hope for, brought a late lunch—burgers, Hershey bars, and cokes from the Officers' Club—for the three to share before the opening of the boxes commenced. After lunch, Mona intuitively understood how Zim wanted to organize the unwrapping ceremony so that Mary didn't turn it into mayhem.

He and Mona cleared two tables. On the first they stacked the packages and boxes. Mary was to stand behind that one. After she revealed each item, Mona was to take it to the second table, arranging like items. *Charm* and other magazines and books in one stack; lipsticks and perfumes in another; snacks, including Gram's mocha cakes, took up the rest of the space. Then came the box of formals, eight of them, and after Mary told Mona the history of each

---

2   Unbeknownst to Mary at the time, her future unit had seen the film *The Nazis Strike* 26 days before she and her fellow nurses watched it.

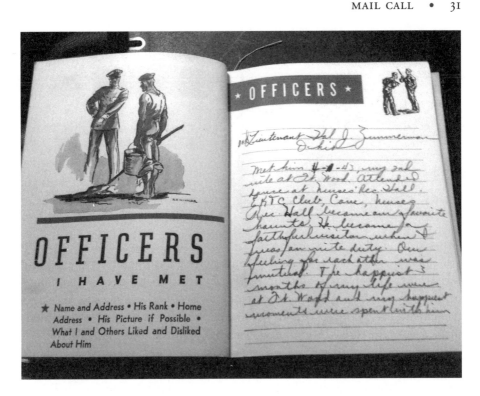

dress, Zim cleared the ash tray and cokes from his table so that Mona could use it to lay out the dresses.

Zim relished Mary's every movement—her "ooos" and "ahhhhs" over every item and the subsequent throwing one aside to look for the next one buried deeper in the box—he loved seeing her so thrilled, enjoyed knowing how much her family must love her. Notwithstanding his mother, this was the first time he'd ever thoroughly enjoyed seeing another person so happy. This was the gal for him. He'd make her his wife before summer. Maybe it was selfish, but he needed to keep her safe from overseas deployment. Marriage was the best option, a method for getting Mary back home to Minnesota as his wife. She would become the woman sending him boxes from now on.

There would be no fear of her losing that beautiful innocence he'd fallen in love with—if he could prevent her from getting any closer to the action. Nursing at Wood was as close as she needed to get to that damn war. If they eloped before he received an alert, then she could become pregnant on a weekend honeymoon and that would be that. She'd receive an honorable discharge as a pregnant married woman. That was his new MO. Mary, a duty to country, in that order.

CHAPTER 5

The Cave

Outside Fort Leonard Wood, close-by private establishments offering anything other than decent burgers and cheap whiskey were few and far between. There was The Cave, a greasy spoon and pub aptly named because of its proximity to a cavern just a hundred feet west of it. Certainly, the restaurant lacked refinement, but patrons came to get drunk, stuff themselves with pub food, then explore the walk-through cave with flashlights and cheerful chatter.

The diner smelled like a cave—dank, musty—but with an overlaying stench of spilled beer. The dining tables, made from soft pine, sheened a sticky wax-like layer, no doubt the result of built-up grease and splashing booze tossed from the rims of crashing mugs.

Lieutenants Lorraine Matzke and Mary Balster entered the establishment with their respective dates, Lieutenants George Francis and Harold Zimmerman. The occasion was Lorraine's birthday. The men decided it was time to elevate the gals' entertainment expectations and get away from the post. The Cave was the most likely choice since none of them had yet experienced it. Twelve weeks into their time at Fort Leonard Wood, there were rumors already that the Air Corps men would be deployed, so time was of the essence to visit The Cave before Lts. Francis and Zimmerman got their marching orders.[1]

A waitress with plump hips and a thoughtful smile led them to a corner table at the rear of the restaurant. She seated the party away from all the fray up front, a reference to the wild throng of drunk enlisted men who crowded

---

1   From Lorraine's recollection, Zim and Fran's first military assignment might have been in Santa Ana, California, where thousands of cadets had arrived for training by March 1942. The cadets lived in tents until the newly formed Army Air Corps base could build housing for the influx of some 5,000 officers who had been sent to train and design the engineering required for war flight.

and bumped their way around the bar. The two gals with their handsome officer dates were certainly too innocent to be exposed to the likes of reprobates. Her assumption was slightly ironic when one considered the poster thumbtacked haphazardly on the wall behind their table, depicting a floozy woman sitting on a soldier's lap. The caption read, "You may think she's just your gal, but she may be everyone's pal."

The poster reminded Mary about the syphilitic patient that she'd seen just a few hours before. For the last few day shifts, she'd been assigned care over the patients newly diagnosed with venereal diseases, one of whom was only 18. He had been admitted to the hospital the day before, convinced that he was suffering from a bad case of the mumps. When his blood serum tests came back positive for syphilis, Mary was charged with breaking the news to him. He said it was impossible. He'd never had sex with a woman, so she promised him that she wouldn't write in his chart that she was compelled to educate him that syphilis could be contracted by having sex with another man. Such documentation would have resulted in his immediate dishonorable discharge. Instead, she assured him that he would recover and make a good soldier. She left his room whispering that one couldn't let such a minor inconvenience get in the way of service to Uncle Sam.[2]

---

2   Patients with severe cases of mumps presented with swollen lymph nodes or salivary glands and a sore throat; however, patients with syphilis could present with these same symptoms.

    In U.S. military hospitals, venereal disease affected one out of eight patients, and before the use of sulfonamides in late 1942, a soldier with venereal disease could not, for all practical purposes, be considered for induction, despite a plea to the War Department from the Director of Selective Service. He argued that a much broader "acceptance of venereals" must be established if the quota of armed services inductees was to be met. The Surgeon General agreed, stating that more syphilitics could be allowed in the service if they could prove to be symptom-free for at least a year. Men with "uncomplicated cases of gonorrhea" would also be considered for induction, but the language of these policies was so broad that an increase in numbers of "venereals" being allowed to serve remained almost nil. But sulfonamides changed the rules almost overnight, so that by the spring of 1943, station hospitals such as Fort Leonard Wood could treat venereal patients and release them for active duty. Army estimates held that over 7,000 men who had been backlogged for a year or more because of a venereal disease diagnosis were treated and released for active duty by March 1943. By 1943's end, 12,000 "venereals" per month were inducted because of the advance of technology surrounding sulfonamides and other new treatments.

    Education for prevention of venereal disease among the armed forces continued to be a priority via countless posters with slogans like, "You can't beat the Axis if you get VD," or "You may think she's just your gal, but she may be everyone's pal." Once patients were diagnosed with VD, education after-the-fact fell to the nurses.

    Fixed Hospitals of the Medical Department (General and Station Hospitals). Technical Manual. The War Department. July 16, 1941.

Once seated, they made a game out of reading aloud the carvings of initials and off-color jokes carved by drunkards into the table's waxy layer. One was hard-pressed to find a virgin spot, but Fran managed, and, with Lorraine, Zim, and Mary as witnesses, he took a steak knife and etched, "HB to LM," as an abbreviation for "Happy Birthday to Lorraine Matzke." Lorraine rewarded him with a kiss on his ample cheek.

Mary thought the carving to be such a sweet gesture that she was motivated to ask Fran a few questions about his own life. It was rare for her to ask about others, even though she truly cared. In social situations she tended toward two opposing behaviors. She struggled to keep up with her own racing thoughts, so to ask someone else in the party about their life was more than she could take on most of the time. If she was the focus of the entertainment, then she could focus. But when others took a conversational lead, she struggled to remain attentive, continually juggling her own thoughts; however, an expression like the one Lt. Francis penned as a way of honoring Lorraine stirred Mary to focus long enough to genuinely become interested in Fran. Though surprised, he was a gregarious sort and was happy to oblige.

He described his upbringing, mid-western just like the others at the table. And like his best buddy Zim, he held an engineering degree and was conscripted to serve in the Army Air Corps. He and Zim had met when they were first stationed in California a few years back.

She listened as attentively as she could muster, but she lost interest in asking him anything else when it became obvious that he didn't seem to know how to describe himself without making references or comparisons to Zim's life. It was a bit odd, as if he only existed as a sidecar to Zim.

Lorraine had noticed it already. She wasn't as beguiling as Mary, but while Mary was often distracted or preoccupied with entertaining a small audience of admirers, Lorraine had time to witness the admirers themselves. She adored Fran, but she hesitated to fall in love with him because he would be leaving the post for overseas duty, sure as the world. And, as Mary noticed tonight, Lorraine already had witnessed his immaturity, that non-stop heralding of Zim as the "be all and end all" of the Army Air Corps. Fran defined himself through Zim's standards. She didn't really find that habit to be attractive, but he had potential. If she could still date him a year from now, she thought a new Lt. Francis would emerge. But she knew the odds of her being in the same place as he would be a year from now were not in the cards. Both these fine men would be gone to war and maybe, just maybe, back home a year from now. The Allies had ripped and roared through Africa. Taking Europe back from Hitler might not take too long at all.

Lorraine loved his looks—the hints of Irish freckles with the opposing olive skin. His mother was Italian, his father Irish. His cheeks reddened when he drank beer, but normally they were a soft, chubby brown. His crew cut didn't allow much in the way of guessing what his hair would be like if he weren't in the service, but the roots looked dark, almost black, close to the color of Mary's. He had a rugged smile, earned through an appealing small gap between the two front teeth. The gals at Fort Leonard Wood thought Lorraine lucky to be dating him, describing him as "a true gem."

Zim, typically quiet and observant, stared into Mary's irises while she forced herself to retain polite eye contact with Fran, although she'd lost interest in his droning at least 10 minutes before. Her eyes stunned Zim the first time they met, but especially now with the tabletop's candle, its burning light shaping her face into a heart and radiating the innermost portions of her irises into a light gray that gave way to a sudden cluster of purples and blues.

He thought it fortunate that Mary's raven locks of hair and stunning eyes could keep him captivated long enough that he could hide his longing for her. It took a soldier's discipline to guard from ogling her buxom figure. She owned 36 inches in the bust and hips. He chuckled when she complained about her "awfully thick Swedish waist." Often, he'd follow with the same reminder, saying that God was going to strike her dead for being so ridiculously self-critical when He'd given her so much.

During the first month they spent together, Mary began to appreciate certain aspects of Zim's looks that she hadn't noticed initially. His teeth were perfectly aligned and boasted a bright white luster. His black and wavy hair was so like Mary's that a few people on post had mistaken them for siblings. In the candlelight, she thought she saw a few gray streaks in his short sideburns, a plus where she was concerned, for as much as she adored Zim's personality, she guiltily found herself wishing that his cheeks and chin would be a bit more sculpted. But the highlights of gray caused by the candle's perfect glow gave his looks that necessary requirement because it provided the possibility that, with age, he'd be more attractive, lose some of that flesh in the face and gain a sophistication that would more readily match his admirable maturity. She adored his winning smile and beautiful manners. Admittedly, she reveled in his attention to her.

There was an unsaid appeal to this night, each of the four intuitively having sensed it. This night would become one to burn in their memories. It was a night of warmth, despite the obnoxious and jolly drunks at the bar. It was a night of innocence, despite Mary's thoughts that she was far more experienced than the waitress could have known. It was a night of stirring sensuality, brought on by their exploration of the cavern after burgers and maybe one too many beers that freed them from inhibition.

Fran coaxed them into the cave exploration. At first, Lorraine protested. It was getting late. She was beginning to feel the exhaustion of a seven-day work week and a heavy meal. But Mary reminded her that they had the next day off, and who knew when they'd be able to get back to this place with their beaus. Lorraine succumbed. Fran paid the tab and handed out the flashlights provided by the restaurant. Off they went.

The cavern's entrance looked like a monster's mouth agape, as if it had been caught yawning when ancient waters formed its shape. A big crowd of frolicking officers were just leaving it. Fran asked them how it was, if it was worth seeing, etc. They wholeheartedly recommended it. They rushed along, their merry voices fading, leaving the four seemingly alone. There was the faint sound of the diner's juke box, but as they trudged deeper into the cavern, all they heard were heavy thumps of dripping water, plopping from the cave's immense ceiling.

The four delighted in the cave's magnificence, oohing and awing their way through halls of wonder, the calcite formations prompting them into a competition. They pointed to a formation, then each took a turn describing what inanimate or animate object that the shape most resembled. But at some point, Fran ventured too far ahead around a dark, unknown turn.

Lorraine called out, but there wasn't any response. Zim wasn't the least bit worried. He reminded Lorraine that Fran flew war planes and knew exactly what risks to take in life. But after a good 10 minutes of calling out to him, Lorraine insisted that they should move faster along the now deep and narrow tunnel. The ceiling had dropped to only a foot and a half above Zim's head, a mere eight or so feet. This cloistering effect caused Lorraine more alarm and frustration because Mary and Zim continued their slow pace, arm in arm, with seemingly no care in the world. She announced to them that she was sorry but was determined to find Fran. Zim gave her the okay. He and Mary would be along shortly, reiterating that Fran was fine, but he understood her concern.

Lorraine fell out of their view, her voice calling, "Fran, where the hell are you? Are you playing a trick on me? It's not funny. I wish you'd answer." For fear of her hearing them, Mary and Zim softly laughed at her silly obsession with having to make sure Fran was okay all the time. Zim whispered that only God knows how the woman's going to react when they're in the throes of air combat in a couple of months.

Under the weight of such a probability, Mary shivered. He felt her shuddering, so he stopped, saying something to the effect that everything would be okay. He found a makeshift niche on which many former visitors had placed candles, evidenced by a prominent pile of cold, melted wax. He took Mary's flashlight along with his own and shut them off. The pitch black of the cave brought immense provocation, as if it were a penetrating, heavy cape that forced such a weight on her she became breathless. She could barely wait for him to touch her.

The pronounced water drops thudding onto the cave floor lessened until she no longer heard the dripping at all. Now there were only the sounds of their own breathing. The anticipation of what was to happen in the next few seconds caused her body to warm. The weight of the pitch-black surroundings held an alluring irony of safety, like the cave was wrapping them in a secret. A series of heightened images of boundless risks now flooded her mind. Suddenly, safety and risk were the same. She closed her eyes to delight in the budding prospects of how he might touch her. Then she heard his hand move along his trousers.

Inside his pocket he searched for the fat candle that had been on their pub table. The weight of it had forced it to fall to the bottom of his pocket. He lit it with his cigarette lighter and allowed it the flirtation of a mere flicker in the niche.

The faint light was just enough. It didn't quell the heavy darkness that had given rise to the anticipation of a sacred and secretive act. The kisses commenced, light and reassuring, then open and intensely freeing, different from the many times they'd kissed before. She didn't know how to describe them to herself. They seemed more intimate but somehow purer.

Then, he charitably moved her to the cave wall, burying his face into her neck. The full weight of his body pressed against her. How his hands were so warm she didn't know. They moved under her dress with perfect knowledge of the places on her body that would give her the most exquisite pleasures. He knew where to touch and how. The efficacy of his movements, the ability to understand where she'd respond with the utmost vulnerability—she knew he must have done this many times, which made her completely trust his experience and instincts.

She was sure many lovers had been here before. Had this been Fran and Zim's plan? Fran to run off, knowing Lorraine would follow, leaving them to find each other and Zim to be left alone with her? The suspicion of such a coordination thrilled her. She thought it calculated but romantic. Then she let go of thoughts altogether and lost all inhibitions. She knew they'd marry. There wasn't any doubt. Zim was the one, but definitely.

But plans for culmination of such a complete submission weren't to be that night. She may have heard something. Was it Lorraine? Yes, it was. She called out, exclaiming that she had found Fran.

Zim pulled his warm hands from her bare skin and fixed her clothing back, but he remained pressed against her until their footsteps sounded very close.

As the four of them made their way back to the cave's opening, present and future thoughts collided. Her head throbbed. She wanted to take in everything that had just happened. She needed to burn the pleasure into a memory strong enough to preclude the passage of time that she knew would try to erase it. She turned the moments with him in that cavern into a time capsule, outlasting what was sure to come—a world without Zim, as war certainly wasn't going to allow them to stay there in that perfect place, nor would it allow Zim to remain at Fort Leonard Wood. She knew all of this.

CHAPTER 6

Hotel Jefferson, St. Louis

In the lobby of the Hotel Jefferson, Camels, Lucky Strikes, and Chesterfields emitted a smog so thick that the GIs pacing the lobby floor looked like sticks colliding in a kettle of bubbling grey soup.

Mary struggled to keep up with Lorraine as the line moved closer to the lobby's check-in desk. She was searching among the contents of a large duffel bag, fumbling in vain to find her pocketbook.

Phew, she thought that she may have left it back at Fort Leonard Wood. But there it was.

Lorraine struck a match to light two Camels. But Mary hesitated.

Standing while smoking made her feel cheap and tawdry. It wasn't a good look for her, and Zim and Inga would not approve. She took two short puffs and handed her Camel back to Lorraine.

To cover her portion of the hotel room expense, Lorraine shoved enough cash in Mary's hand and waddled off to find somewhere to perch. Her ankle was on fire with pain. She grabbed the corner edge of a long sofa, fully occupied with other nurses. She paid no mind to the few of them who stared at her while she smoked both cigarettes, methodically taking a deep drag on each.

Along with Mary and Lorraine, several nurses from Fort Leonard Wood had received the two-day pass. There were so many familiar faces from the post that the two wondered who might be left to take care of the patient load. Maybe the new chief nurse wasn't that stellar after all. Her scheduling seemed to be a bit off.

Zim and Fran were to arrive later that afternoon, but since the four spent so much time together at the post, Zim had insisted that Lorraine and Fran make their own plans. He needed to spend time with Mary alone. They all speculated that since it was almost the first week of July already, it would be a matter of weeks, if not days, until the men would receive orders overseas.

Lorraine limped toward the elevator with Mary. Their hotel room was lovely, but before they did anything else, Mary insisted that Lorraine lie on a chaise lounge by the window. She needed to get a good look at that ankle in the light.

Lorraine's right ankle had borne the brunt of too many requisite hikes in the sludge. She wondered if she was fit for this army life.

Not that Mary was cut out for it, either. She didn't give two hoots for those hikes, had no appreciation or understanding of their purpose, especially when one considered Lorraine's injury. Why didn't the chief realize that probably all of them would end up getting injuries from those darn hikes? Then no one would be able to take care of the boys. Honestly, the army was so exasperating at times.

She asked Lorraine to describe the pain level of that ankle. It wasn't great, but at least it wasn't intolerable, not compared to the way it looked. Both were hoping that it was simply an acute injury and not something chronic.

Mary wanted to call the bellman. Maybe he could bring up some ice to reduce the swelling.

Lorraine didn't argue. She had wanted to pal around with Mary at The Famous-Barr for the afternoon.[1] They planned to shop a bit and then get their hair done. But she'd cancel and ice the ankle. That was the prudent thing to do.

Mary wouldn't be more than a couple of hours and when she returned, she'd draw Lorraine a nice hot bath.

Soon the bellman came, and Mary sat at the end of the chaise to hold the bag of ice on the swelling. Lorraine asked her if she'd noticed that new nurse in the lobby, the one who'd been stationed at Boca prior to her arrival at Fort Leonard Wood.

Yes, she'd noticed but didn't feel like chewing the fat with her. She didn't want to ruin her two-day leave thinking about that rotten deal.

The nurse had known Clinton. He'd been a patient of hers when he'd had that eye infection back in April. In May, she was transferred to Fort Leonard Wood and worked her first shift with Mary. During small talk, she asked Mary where she grew up. When Mary said St. Paul, she said that she'd had a patient from St. Paul just a few weeks before in Boca.

Funny, Mary had said, and then explained that her boyfriend was a patient on Medical Ward down in Boca. He'd been in for a nasty eye infection.

Perplexed, the gal said that Mary's beau couldn't be the same as her patient after all, although he was also in for an eye infection. The lieutenant that she'd

---

1   The Famous-Barr was another department store in St. Louis during the golden age of department stores.

cared for was dating a buxom blonde who worked on the Surgical Ward. She was a faithful daily visitor. What a coincidence.

Coincidental as it was, Lorraine said, it was fortuitous. After all, Mary had to admit that the nurse's accidental revelation that Clinton was a two-timer let Mary off the hook from breaking it off with him. How could Mary consider that such a raw deal? It was a perfect way to end things with Clinton. Mary came out smelling like a rose when, in fact, she'd fallen for Zim anyway, so what did it matter if Clinton had moved on, too?

It was just the principle of the thing. He hadn't been honest. He'd pretended that the eye infection was so bad that his visit to Fort Leonard Wood to see Mary would need to be postponed when really it was because he had a new girlfriend that somehow, he'd failed to mention in every phone call. Thank God, she hadn't married him last year right after he was conscripted. They'd talked about it on more than one occasion. That would have been disastrous.

***

On the walk back to the Jefferson from The Famous-Barr, she thought about the evening's plans with Zim. Should she tell him that she was thinking about signing up for foreign duty? He'd have a darn fit, but what else was she to do? Stay at Fort Leonard Wood for the duration and sit on pins and needles while Zim risked his life and their future? She'd rather be in the thick of it, too. At least that way she'd be so busy she wouldn't have time to think, and she'd feel a lot more useful. And she'd know more what Zim was going through if she was going through something similar. Probably shouldn't say that to him, though. He'd say that was the most asinine thing he'd ever heard. She knew him.

She'd play it by ear. Let him dominate the conversation for once. Not that he would. He seemed to prefer staring at her while she did the talking. Not that she minded. She adored being adored. That she had to admit.

***

At 7:15 p.m., she meandered through the formal dining room of the Hotel Jefferson, following the host to Zim's table. She wore black sling backs and an off-the-shoulder red gown with black tendrils falling from a tightly drawn waist. Her clutch, a hand-woven mesh of pearls and gold beads, dangled under her left hand, supported by gold chains crossing over her chest. It was reminiscent of the flapper look, and, indeed, the purse had been Inga's, not that she would have ever bought it. Her father had given it to her mother, his extravagance always bestowed on the women of his life—Inga, Mary, Nancy, and Constance.

They talked about the dessert banquet table. Someone at the hotel had meticulously set it to resemble a French village, that is, a French village before the Nazis' pillages. Candles served to symbolize streetlights, cakes were made to look like a town's quaint buildings, the fondant icing was layered to look like red and pink bricks. Brown icing formed on top of the cakes to suggest slate and tile roofing and drops of white frosting pressed and piled against chimneys to hint at the gathering of snow. Pastries formed lines and curves to resemble a street, and trees were made from stacked cookies with bits of cherries and nuts randomly placed on them to suggest buds and blooms.

"Clever," Zim said.

So typical of a man, Mary thought, especially an engineer. Romantic scenery was lost on him, but she appreciated his attempts at romance. After all, he'd planned the evening so well. And he'd insisted they dine alone. And, as always, his dancing was wildly stunning and graceful. A Fred Astaire, no doubt.

But they didn't dance much that night. He preferred staring at her, as if he needed to drink her in.

Although she'd planned to allow him the lead in conversation, his mood was tempered. She couldn't read him. Did he know something she didn't? Maybe he'd received orders and was waiting until the end of the night to tell her. She stuck to her plan to be quiet, despite his reticence to talk.

Although she wasn't aware of it then, those hours spent with Zim that evening melted into a memory that would emerge 16 months later in a country far from home with a man who would not be Zim.

***

War is one of those heightened times in human experience that mixes memory with consciousness and creates something outside of space and time. Its power warps constants. In war, memory becomes a type of consciousness, a thing in and of itself.

She couldn't have known this that night. Soon, though, it would become clear to her just how murky the past, present, and future could be.

War's power was unspeakable, its timelessness unbearable. Soon, her life, more so than Zim's, would change dramatically. And the change would begin in less than 12 hours.

CHAPTER 7

Please Forgive This Depressing Missive

Mary hadn't been able to fall into a deep asleep until around 4 in the morning, her mind reeling about all the comments Zim had made the night before about their future, mostly during dessert and afterwards, when they strolled around the lobby and outdoors for a couple of hours. She'd promised herself to be quiet and, for the most part, she had held to it. She did fall off the no-talking wagon when he said that she was "absolutely regal." She felt uncomfortable with those kinds of compliments, so at that point, she commenced to the yacking.

Then he placed his hand over her mouth gently. He smiled at her. They laughed because she admitted to him that she'd promised herself earlier to be quiet that night. Then he said that it seemed to him that sometimes she talked incessantly to detract from her allure. And, honestly, he said, it did. He asked her why she often took to the chattering during intimate moments or when he was commenting about her beauty. She didn't know, but she really appreciated the compliments and was so happy that she looked pretty to him. She'd try to do better accepting his admiration. Then he said he was glad, as the next time they were awarded a two-day leave, he wanted to arrange for them to have engagement photographs taken. She mulled over those words during that restless night. Her knowledge about Zim's personality opposed the idea that he was simply caught up in the night's romantic ambience. Zim was quite serious and level-headed. He never made impulsive decisions. But she worried. She chastised herself for being worried, but she couldn't help it. She should be happy. She was, no doubt, so happy. But something was nagging her. She didn't know what it was. She was head over heels in love with Zim, so why worry?

Finally, she talked herself into settling down. She and Zim would figure everything out, she assured herself. Then she fell asleep and awoke to the sharp ring of the hotel room's telephone. Lorraine answered it. Mary sat up in a bit of a fog but heard Lorraine say something like, "Oh, golly. Okay.

Okay. We'll hurry." Later, Mary and Lorraine agreed that they'd never received a phone call so brief but so powerful in its message. They had been relieved of duty from Fort Leonard Wood. They had less than an hour to pack, check out of the hotel, and jump on the bus to Ft. Leonard Wood, and would receive new orders once they were back at the post. They packed like "bats out of hell," Mary said. Then, hurriedly, she penned a quick note of explanation to Zim and shoved it under his hotel room door on the way to the lobby to catch the bus.

It was 140 miles from St. Louis to Ft. Leonard Wood, so during the bus ride, Mary and Lorraine attempted to sort through the little information they had. A few gals in the lobby told them that they heard she, Lorraine, and a few other gals were headed to maneuvers, but they weren't sure where. "Oh, the irony," Mary said to Lorraine. "All this time we thought for sure that Zim and Francis would be the ones receiving orders to leave good ole Ft. Wood, but it was us who received them."

> July 4, 1943
> Dearest Mom, Dad, and all,
>
> It's 7 A.M. this fourth of July, 1943, and I'm about to set out on a new venture. By the time you receive this you will have heard the news and don't know as I can add much to it at this time but decided I must send off one last letter from Ft. Wood. Our orders came Fri. A.M. and we were relieved of duty immediately and have been in a daze ever since. Have no idea what the future holds but the most authentic report is that we're to set up an evacuation hospital somewhere around Shelbyville, Tennessee, where maneuvers are starting now and no doubt will continue throughout the summer. It's about 600 miles from here. Leave at noon today arriving in St. Louis at 6 where we have a four hour stop over. Plan to eat dinner there and relax. Have lower Pullmans from there to Nashville. Expect to arrive at our destination about 3 tomorrow.
>
> You can imagine the time we've had getting packed. Had to add a foot locker and another bag to my luggage. Am also shipping a lot of stuff home which I will tell you about later. Only hope it arrives safely. If it hadn't been for Zim, wouldn't be packed yet. He organized my packing beautifully and has been such a wonderful help these last two days.
>
> Every available minute I've spent with Zim. Last nite we went to the ERTO informal dance. They had the dance floor on the tennis courts which was surrounded by tables. At 2 A.M. decided to take a plunge in the pool which we did, and it was wonderful. Got back here at 4 and turned in at 5 so guess I'll be catching up on my shuteye on the train. Of course Zim and I plan to get together after the war but you know how that will probably turn out. Time and distance will probably thwart any plans we have now. Well, I came into the ANC to do my part and duty will have to come 1st and I'll worry about the rest later. Lorraine and I have been crying so much the last few hours but have reconciled ourselves to the fact now that we are no longer master of our fate at least for the duration and guess the experience we will get will be valuable in the years to come.

The unit that Mary, Lorraine, and Mona joined had been formed in August 1942 at Camp Atterbury, Indiana, and at that time was newly named the

"39th Evacuation Hospital." The unit's commander, Lieutenant Colonel Allen N. Bracher, had been charged with command over all personnel, both officers and enlisted men, who'd either received on-the-job training in first aid, triage, and injury evacuation protocols or who had attended medic training in Washington, D.C. From August 1942 until June 1943, the men of this unit knew that nurses would be joining them to train for overseas service. But the nurses who would eventually join them had no idea; that is, until they were given a mere two-day notice that they would become members of the 39th Evacuation Hospital. The male members of the unit had long anticipated the nurses' arrival and were already set up on maneuvers in middle Tennessee.[1]

July 6, 1943
Dearest Everyone,
    Greetings from your GI maiden who is now strictly GI and who is in the 2nd scene, act one of her life in the ANC. This scene opened when she left dear old Ft. Wood Sunday July 4th that noon embarking for parts unknown full of anticipation, bewilderment and perhaps a little fear. Left Nashville at noon yesterday and after getting off the train at a funny little Southern town, Wartrace, immediately went to a gov't-approved restaurant—there was one in the town, she and 12 other nurses sat in a jeep until 5 p.m. waiting for transportation to the 39th Evacuation Hospital, which is located in some cow pasture in this maneuver area, I can't say just where. Our transportation came in the form of a two-ton government truck, one of those covered wagon affairs. The signal corps treated us royally by first taking us up to their quarters where we had some very good chow and a sack of oranges and apples as a gift. We all piled in the truck again and were taken about 20 miles down some horribly dusty road arriving in one piece with gray hair and very bedraggled looking. We were immediately assigned to tents—4 girls to a tent and our chief nurse chose to bunk with us until she gets her own tent where she will have her office. We were then given bed rolls in which we discovered a gas mask, flashlight, mess kit, mosquito netting, blankets, canteen, 1st aid kit and helmets which are in two part[s], the inside plastic part that we wear at all times along with our gas mask as at any time we may expect an attack as active maneuvers are in progress The outside of our helmets, the iron part, we use for everything from soup to nuts. When we finish these letters plan to wash our clothes in them. We were in bed by 9:30 last nite and had a wonderful nite's sleep except for one interruption when a storm came up and we had to let down our tent flaps. We undress by flashlite as we don't have lanterns or candles—electric lights? Who ever heard of them? Reveille is at 5:45, we must go to breakfast between 6:30 and 7. We place our mess kits in a huge pot of boiling water before we line up for chow which this morning consisted of french toast, bacon, and coffee. When we finish, we scrape our kits, place them 1st in a pot of boiling soap water, then 2 rinsing waters which are kept at boiling temperature at all times. Our chief is going to Camp Forrest this morning where the station hospital is located, and get our fatigues, high topped shoes, and trench coats. We won't go on duty until we have our fatigues which are in the form of coveralls. We'll be some glamour girls by the time this is over. Have no idea how long maneuvers will last or how long we will be here. This 39th Evac. Hosp. is

1   Camp Atterbury, Indiana, 39th Evacuation Hospital, Daily Log. 30 August 1942–14 November 1945, declassified, Authority 735017 by: SJ, NARA, January 21, 2001.

what is known as a semi-mobile unit. It is divided into Echelons A and B—must be able to move nearer the front or vice versa. Our chief nurse is just leaving for town all dressed up in helmet, gas mask, skirt, and shirt. Our luggage hasn't arrived as yet, and when it does you may expect a couple of bags of clothes arriving at 1262, I hope. The girls at Ft. Wood promised to see that our cardboard boxes got off OK. Intend to keep only my footlocker and small bag as we have to move at a moment's notice and when we do get sent back to a station hospital or wherever we go will have to send for them. We weren't told what we were getting into so of course brought a million things we won't use including white uniforms, etc. Know I owe money again and will take care of it as soon as we receive transportation reimbursement which should be about $30. Have the rest of my money in travelers checks which is the safest at a place like this, I guess. This hosp. is laid out in the form of a cross, and everything is identical with an overseas setup. We are subject to attack at any time by the red army (the red and blue are fighting here) and so will dig our own slit trenches and be able to crawl into them at a moment's notice.

Don't dare think of Ft. Wood and the paradise I left behind. Doubt I will ever have such happy times again. We are mostly young nurses here—there will be 20 of us when the unit is complete. The life is going to be rugged and don't know just how we'll emerge from it, but it will be a very valuable experience and good preparation for foreign duty in case we do get sent. However, there is a new A.R. out which states that we must have leaves before going to a P.E. and besides doubt if we ever will go—it depends upon how this unit clicks, etc.[2]

Could go on for hours but as usual time is precious—we must make good use of our daylight as flashlights aren't too good for letter writing, etc.

Will close now with all my love to all of you.

Please address my letters as follows:

2nd Lt. M. E. Balster, ANC N775512

39th Evacuation Hospital

APO #402

Nashville, Tennessee

c/o Postmaster

On the train from Nashville to Wartrace, Mona sat next to Mary. Both wrote in their service diaries. Then to pass the time, they let each other read what they'd written.

Mona pointed to one of Mary's entries and said, "Oh, Mary. Golly, I know it's so hard." Mary had written, "the best three months of my life were spent at good ole Fort Leonard Wood, and the best moments were spent with Zim." Mona figured that the odds were against Mary and Zim. It was probable that they'd never see each other again.

***

At their first briefing, Major Scanlon spoke first. His demeanor held the usual authoritative air of a commanding officer, but the nursing staff sensed there

2   AR: Army Regulation; PE or POE: point of embarkation.

was also a kindness to him. He seemed to be a strong leader, comfortable with his role, and yet not at all pompous. Even his lean body shape matched Mary's ideal of a man in charge. She thought that if a stranger were to walk in at that point, he would have guessed that Scanlon was the boss. But she was wrong. He wasn't the highest-ranking officer there.

The next man up was the big guy in charge, Col. Allen N. Bracher. He gave the formal welcome. He had a fuller face and looked younger than the major, but she didn't think that could be possible, given their difference in rank. He wore a thin mustache that helped to add a bit of sophistication to him, but even with the mustache and insignia, he still appeared younger than Major Scanlon. She found out later that Col. Bracher was 37, Scanlon, 33. The major looked about 45 but that was probably due to this thin frame that hadn't allowed any facial fat. In comparison to his boss, the major's fair skin aged him, too, along with his poor eyesight. He was never without his gold-rimmed glasses that framed big, blinking brown eyes.

Col. Bracher expressed his deepest admiration for the new crop of nurses, reiterating that the army was indebted to all of them for the contributions they were making to the war effort. Then he made what the nurses realized was an inside joke, something about when he and his men were on maneuvers close to Camp Atterbury, Indiana, they found out the hard way how difficult it was to care for patients in the field without nurses' expertise. His comments helped the nurses' morale, but it was short-lived, as dysentery soon overwhelmed the camp and carried that unique ability of dissolving any former pride that belonged with serving as an evac nurse.

Last up was Chief Maxson. She planned to run 11-hour shifts to allow time for the nurses to become inured to outdoor living. Day shift would run from 0700 until 1800. The night shift would run from 1900 until 0600. Corpsmen would cover the twelfth hour for each shift and would contact a nurse if something emergent arose. Medical Wards would consist of two tents, one for officers, the other for enlisted personnel.

July 9, 1943
Dearest Family,

It's 1 p.m. and four of us are sitting on a blanket in our bathing suits in the bright sunlite. Have to go back on duty at 3 and heaven knows when I'll get off. We're working hard, our morale is very low, and everyone is ready to go AWOL. The hospital is not organized, living conditions are about as rugged as they could possibly be, and we're all wondering how we can endure it until Sept. when maneuvers should be over. Hope to go back to a station hospital then—none of us signed up for foreign duty and now I know for sure I don't want any part of it, but if they send us anyway guess we'll take it and like it. Think we will get leaves after maneuvers and that's the only thing we're living for now. As this is a mobile unit,

7-8-43   9 P.M.   by flashlite
Utterly Scene - sitting on cot
in tent located in home
cow pasture near Shelbyville, Te.

Utterly exhausted - our morale
is low - duty very discouraging
as hospital is not organized.
Too tired to write any more.

7-10-43
8 P.M. - Two lonely, discouraged
nurses sitting on a foot locker in
tent door thinking hell would
have nothing on the way we
feel. To top off our discontent
and discouragement the old GI
dysentery bug grabbed us, and
we haven't strength enough to do
anything but go to bed, which is
where we'll both be in a very

short while as it's getting too
dark to see and we must conserve
our flashlite batteries.
We feel like hell — splitting
headaches, nausea, vomiting,
horrible back aches, lethargy
and utterly worn out from our
frequent walks to the little house
that begins with L. Treatment
consists of sulfaguanadine q4h
and now we are trying to decide
which is worse — the disease or
the cure.
Our only comfort is each other's
presence — we laugh together,
cry together and gripe together — hell
or high water won't separate us if
we can help it. Our bodies are
here but our hearts are back at
dear old Ft. Wood = the two best
shavetails in the U.S. Army. How
can I endure this life for 3 months?...

Just draw on your grit; it's so easy to quit—
It's the keeping your chin up that's hard.—Robert W. Service

The less there is of fear, the less there is of danger.

we move to another cow pasture about once a week between problems. Therefore, you can expect my bags to arrive sometime next week, and you can leave them packed as will need the stuff again when I get back to civilization. We are allowed to go to town once a week, but only 5 of us can leave at one time. Must be back by midnight or the MP's will pick us up. As there are no decent towns around here, and nothing to do when you get there, we would just as soon stick around here, and we're so tired we don't care to put on those hot old GI uniforms anyway. We are paying double for those happy days at Ft. Wood. I start to cry every time I think of Zim and all the other wonderful people I left behind. No other man will ever mean anything to me after knowing him. We talked of marriage but realized how utterly foolish it would have been with me in the ANC as after all I made a contract with Uncle Sam and intend to keep it no matter what. Besides, it would be a thousand times worse being separated from him if we were married. Separation, war, etc., make the odds too great to expect anything from the future so I just don't anymore.

Realize this is a terrible letter but just can't help it. All 20 of us feel the same way—in fact the whole outfit is low.

Lorraine is quite sick—the first of our bunch to get dysentery which is the main complaint around here. It's awful stuff but doesn't last long.

It gets cold here at nite, and we sleep under mosquito netting as this is malaria country—no sheets or pillows but manage to rest well anyway. It's rather pretty around here—our pasture is surrounded by hills and trees. Wear our fatigues all the time with anklets and saddle shoes until our high-top ones arrive. Wear our rank on our collar, a blue band on our left shoulder as we belong to the blue army and a #2 on our left sleeve for 2nd army. I have two tent wards—one is the officer's ward where I have to spend more time as even out in the field, they expect more than the enlisted men.

So help me if anyone ever asks me to go on a picnic again, their name will be mud. I'm going to live in a glass house where I can enjoy nature from the inside and sleep all day on a Beautyrest mattress. There's going to be an outdoor movie (don't know where else it could be). They're going to rig up some showers for us from the creek and nurses' hours are between 2 and 4 and it's 2 now so guess we'll truck over—it's the best part of the day for us even if the water is quite cool, we have the sky for a roof and a few men hanging around right outside the canvas—for protection I imagine.

Please forgive this depressing missive. Hope the next one will be to a different tune…

By nightfall July 9, Mary, Mona, and many other nurses joined in Lorraine's misery with their first bout of dysentery. The sole therapy for it was to gulp "sulfa-guanidine" every four hours and to resist regurgitation right after ingesting the medicine, even though the stuff was so foul and metallic that a mouthful of vomit would have been a more welcome taste.

If dysentery was first on the list of greatest nuisances, then second on that list were the insects, especially black flies, and malaria mosquitoes.[3] The fly population became so fierce by mid-July that there weren't enough cow paddies from which the flies could feed, so they chose to land on the faces and hands of the 39th.

July 11, 1943
Dearest Family,

Just a few lines before I hit the old bunk again. It's 8:30 P.M. and dark as pitch so am writing by flashlite again.

Received the dress, etc. this P.M. and had to pack it right back up again crying while I did it. Put it in with Lorraine's baggage as there wasn't any room left in mine. Have several other things in her bag also so if you will stop over at Matzke's and collect it will appreciate it. Have to send our baggage collect but plan to send $100 home as soon as I get my check so that should cover the expenses that have been mounting up and that I have been burdening you with. The only good thing about this deal is that it will be easy on the pocketbook. On top of our other sorrows half of us fell victim to the old GI dysentery bug this week. Haven't eaten for 3 days and am so weak, haven't hardly strength to comb my hair. We've been taking sulphaguanidine every 4 hrs. which is almost worse than the disease. This dysentery is accompanied by severe headache, backache, cramps, and lethargy. All I want to do is sleep. Feel better tonite, tho, and plan to go back to work tomorrow. If this life is a sample of foreign duty, we want no part of it and have made up our minds that no matter what they do to us we won't go across the pond as can see now that we wouldn't be worth a darn if we ever did get back. Between flies and numerous other insects, no warm weather or water, no lights, and a very depressed state of mind we are all just about nuts and can't see how we can possibly endure this life until fall. The nites are damp and cold, the days hot and sticky. There is nothing to look forward to—have discovered that they could get along very well without nurses here as the corpsmen do all the actual nursing care and all we can figure out is that we were sent here to boost morale which seems impossible the

---

3   "Malaria mosquitoes" is a reference to mosquitoes that carried malaria. The diseased mosquitoes weren't eradicated with DDT in the United States until the 1950s.

way we feel now. This is no life for a girl and would give anything if I was a civilian again or back at Ft. Wood.

We move at the end of the week, and I hate to think of it.

Our only prayer now is that we'll get leaves when this is over and then get back to a station hospital.

Will send the keys to my luggage this week so you can take the stuff out and then I'll repack it when I get home. Am living for the day when I can put on a white uniform again and some pretty clothes. Think my civies will still fit as it's a cinch I'll never put on weight here.

We don't ever see a newspaper or hear a radio so have no idea what the world news is but pray that it's encouraging and hope that the day isn't too far distant when we can start living again.

Please forgive these awful letters—know I shouldn't be writing to you this way but maybe the next one will be more cheerful.

Hope you are all well. I miss you all so much. Please write often as that's all I have to look forward to now.

I think I have some conception now of what our boys and girls are going thru over there and realize that it's a thousand times worse with constant fear prevailing. We are living exactly as if we were over there, tho,—can't even hang our clothes outside as we are supposed to practice camouflage at all times. You can imagine what condition they'll be in when I get back to civilization—washing them in cold water and hanging them in dark tents to dry.

Well, better I should fix my mosquito netting and chase the spiders etc., out of my bed so I can go to sleep in peace. Last nite killed a black widow spider and two other malaria mosquitoes.

Must close now,

All my love to the best family a gal ever had—would give anything if I was home with you. Guess I'm just a sissy but s'pose I'll get hardened to it after a while.

Love, Mary

For Mary, there were two reprieves from the misery. The first was in the form of a letter from Zim. He confessed that he hadn't told her the entirety of his plans for their future. Apparently, the professional engagement photos were only part of the plan. He'd also planned for them to elope the next time they had the opportunity to take leave for St. Louis. Although it wasn't to be, his letter offered Mary hope that one day they would have their future. The fantasy of an impending happy marriage to Zim helped her through many of those first miserable days of maneuvers.

The other reprieve was a one-night leave with Mona, Lorraine, and a few other nurses. They climbed into a weapons carrier along with seven male officers for a 50-mile rough ride into Nashville. Mary bought a mirror for the tent, and they all got pillows and candles at Harvey's Department Store, a new fun place to shop that included screaming monkeys, a huge lunch counter, even escalators that featured carousel horses.

Upon their return to the post, as they had come to expect, they were to pack up and make ready to be moved, this time closer to a town called Shelbyville and further away from Nashville. They would become the "Red Army" as opposed to having been the "Blue Army." They hunted for their red ribbons that were worn on their left shoulders and donned their overseas caps for the "new problem," a maneuvers expression that basically meant that soldiers were being ordered to experience a new hypothetical war simulation.

The cow pasture was replaced with more "woodsy" environs. Instead of broadleaf and sedges, crab grasses and rag weed, they contended with ferns and mildew, chiggers, and wood ticks. Even though their clothes never felt dry once they arrived at their new area, they were happy to get out of the sun-drenched open fields. During those cow pasture days, there had been no shade for the lyster bag so the water from it had taken on the sun's heat. Consequently, the gals were chronically thirsty because the water was so hot that when they attempted to drink it, they would experience a wave of nausea. The lyster bag was now shaded by swamp oaks and cypress trees, so the water was far more quenching.

The nurses' convoy arrived at the new area just in time to see the hospital, library, and PX tents go up in a field and watch how the corpsmen arranged them in the form of a cross. Everyone was ordered to start digging their foxholes again, and all were happy that their living quarter tents were arranged in the dense woods where soft, fertile creek dirt would provide a less burdensome dig. As Mary and Lorraine began to dig their respective fox holes, their conversation carried a more positive tone than they'd been able to muster since their last days at Ft. Wood, one saying to the other that wasn't it just marvelous that they'd figured out how to wash and rinse their thick heads of hair in their helmets instead of depending on the showers that only offered a trickle from lack of water pressure.

Even the dense air didn't bother them. They chirped and trilled like two little titmice as whipping winds cooled them while they dug. When they were halfway finished, they acknowledged that the distant thunder was not so distant anymore and assured each other that the following morning would offer a more efficient dig once the impending rain softened the earth.

A stray cat also aided in their morale boost. It had shown up and instantly became an object of affection for Mona and Lorraine. Even though Mary was allergic to cats, she loved her from a distance and named her "Nikki."

Since they'd been on maneuvers, Mary, Mona, and Lorraine had not enjoyed the comfort of a pillow. They couldn't wait to sleep on them their first night in the new maneuver area. It turned out to be the only night Mary slept on hers. Even though the 39th had $60,000 worth of beautiful surgical instruments and plenty of other good equipment, no one, not even patients, was issued a pillow:

> Am now in charge of officer's ward and a surgical ward so have been really doing some nursing this past week. Yesterday they did an emergency appendectomy on a 1st Lt. and of course he's under my care. Tonite he is sleeping on my pillow as they don't have any pillows here and those cots are no fun for a post-operative pt. His appendix was ruptured, and he just about went out on them in surgery, but he's doing wonderfully today. This P.M. I gave him a bath and alcohol rub. Heated the water on my little oil stove in my surgical ward and knelt on the ground to bathe him. Yes, we are doing our nursing under rugged conditions and doing things the hard way but I'm not griping about our work. It's this messy living, washing in cold water, never having any place to put our things, looking like a mess all the time and restricted living that's hard to take…

The rain was defying gravity and pelleting through the air horizontally, so she took up one patient's offer to borrow his trench coat. Hers had been issued at Fort Leonard Wood, but it had been far too big, so Chief Maxson had ordered her to drop it off at the tailor's before they left Missouri. But the trench coat still hadn't caught up to her on maneuvers.

Since she now sported a trench coat, she just had to stop by the PX before heading to the tent. She had a hankering for a coke and a Hershey bar.

Living quarter tents were half an acre away, set up against a tree line that marked the beginnings of a deep, thick forest. It was nice to be closer to the showers, although they were still about a half-acre away down a trail that the corpsmen had cut through canebrakes.

She grabbed six Hershey bars and five Coca-Cola bottles. The PX only offered a paper sack to place her items in, and that certainly would not hold up in the deluge of rain that pounded on top of the PX tent. She took off her helmet, stuffed the chocolate bars inside the plastic part, and placed it back on her head. She stuck two coke bottles in each side pocket and carried the one that she asked for them to open there. She hadn't been able to quench her thirst all evening.

She left the PX tent looking like a grey wet ghost chugging down a Coca-Cola. With a quick but awkward pace, she made it through the grassy field and began the trek down toward the forest. The rain had come so fast that it had already eroded the dirt floor of the woods and had turned the entire trail to the tents into thick, stubborn goo. At the tent entrance, she plopped down on a crate and attempted to get the high-tops off. She belched, surprising

Mona and Lorraine. Mary may have been rebellious in some ways, but she never burped out loud.

High-tops removed, she began crawling around in her space, peeking under her bedroll, looking frustrated and anxious, telling Lorraine that she was searching for the can opener to offer Nikki the cat a can of chicken because she'd heard her meowing.

The rain was not as loud as it had been a few minutes earlier, but darkness fell over them so suddenly that Mona grabbed for her flashlight so that she could see to light a few candles.

In the light, Lorraine noticed Mary's face. It looked ruddy and flushed. She looked like she might be getting sick.

Mary opened the cooked chicken and plopped it down in a small tin plate for Nikki. When she peered down at her muddy pants' legs, she felt saliva filling up her mouth. Her ears started ringing, and all her nerve endings tingled. Acid coated her throat. She barely made it to the tent opening and began vomiting with brute force, her bottom still inside the tent.

Then she disappeared altogether. Lorraine and Mona knew that she didn't have a flashlight on her and that she wasn't wearing any shoes. Mona held a flashlight in one hand and a candle in the other for Lorraine to search for her own shoes and trench coat. They knew that despite the storm, Mary was headed for the showers.

Despite her large size, Lorraine moved quickly when required. She left Mona in the tent to tend to Mary's muddy shoes and followed the trail to the creek.[4]

The storm howled with fury, but Lorraine and Mary hardly noticed. Lorraine helped free Mary from the soiled navy pants and then reached over her to pull the string that the engineers had installed to operate the shower faucet. Mary scrubbed herself with a rough rag that Lorraine had hurriedly stuffed in her own trench coat. Then Mary attempted to rinse out her uniform, but another bout of harsh lower abdominal pain overtook her.

"Oh, God, Lorraine, I'm so sick."

This second bout of dysentery seemed far worse than the one they'd all gone through only two weeks earlier.

---

4   Interview, Lorraine Matzke, Spokane, WA, 1978.

CHAPTER 8

No Excuses

Lt. Elizabeth O'Reilly showed up in August, replacing a gal who'd been dishonorably discharged for sitting on a cot with an enlisted man. Lt. O'Reilly was lanky-tall, looked a bit boyish, and wasn't at all voluptuous. But she was divine.

She was the first southerner in Mary's life who contradicted every notion Mary ever held previously about southerners. That there could exist such a fine specimen of class from the Deep South, why, it just didn't seem possible. These people were lazy, poor, had nothing in the way of modern conveniences, heck, many didn't even have indoor plumbing for goodness' sake, and their farms were just completely littered with worn-out cars that were propped up with boards and concrete blocks and what have you. Whoever heard of actual tires? The tires never seemed to be attached to axles; instead, they were usually abandoned in fields. Weeds and moccasin snakes and malaria mosquitoes used them to hatch their eggs. Sometimes tires hung from trees by ropes that served as children's swings. The poor babies never saw a proper swing set. Parks? Non-existent.

Elizabeth arrived at a most inopportune time. Chief Maxson had just announced that they would be increasing their 5-mile hike to an 8-mile. But this gal Elizabeth just smiled and said everything was gonna be alright. How she could own such an attitude was beyond Mary and Lorraine. They agreed to just give her time. She'd find out first-hand the misery they'd come to expect each day.

The bucolic scenery wasn't lost on them, the topography of hills, the myriad varieties of oaks and hickory trees that were middle Tennessee. But it was during the hikes that the nurses witnessed abject poverty. It was disturbing, as if the Depression had lingered and become a part of the landscape.

On the 8-mile, the nurses heard what sounded like a Motorola radio blaring. They reached a low-lying field and marched by some rusted farm equipment and a Bonnie and Clyde-looking car. Some poor fellow had fallen asleep inside. Elizabeth said it was common for the poor to rig up a radio inside a non-working car, probably to escape all the screaming children running around the shacks.

Mary didn't know how the radio was running. She guessed the battery still somehow worked in the jalopy, but she was certain that gas hadn't run through it in probably over a decade. And now, in contrast to all the squalor and backwardness, there was this paragon of nobility from Birmingham, Alabama, Lt. Elizabeth O' Reilly, explaining the plight of the poor but obviously only as an observer. Some parts of the South must be better off economically than middle Tennessee. Elizabeth didn't fit the mold of the stereotypical southerner that Mary had witnessed so far. That was certain.

Chiefee asked Mona to work alongside Elizabeth during her first couple of shifts. Soon after, Mary worked with her, agreed with Mona that her skills were excellent, adding that her grace extended to her bedside manner. She was a keeper. Within a week of Elizabeth's arrival, one of the patients labeled her with a nickname that everyone in the unit immediately took to. He called her "Alabama." From that week on, no one ever called her Elizabeth again. Alabama it was. Alabama it would always be.

Ever since their arrival in Tennessee, the nurses had made a game of mimicking accents. When Alabama arrived, hers became the instant favorite. Mary practiced in vain to imitate it, and Alabama reprised, "Mary, you are so darlin' of a puhson all on your own. No need at all to mimic me."

Sometime during late August or early September, new fatigues and wool leggings arrived. Mary, Alabama, Mona, and Lorraine reserved 30 minutes prior to chow one evening to try on their newest army attire. The leggings were, in a word, dreadful. They were hot, itchy, and it made no sense to wear wool in the humid climate. In addition, they were the "one size fits all" type. Lorraine and Mona's were too snug, and Alabama's far too short. Mary's fit "okay" but later someone noticed that she'd put hers on backwards, so, admittedly, they did fit her "pretty well" once she put them on correctly. But with the temperature at least 90 degrees inside the tent, and with the leggings on, they sweated so profusely that they had to lie down on their cots to peel them off their damp skin. The gals made the unanimous decision that Mary should be the voice of protest regarding the leggings. However, a complaint should go up the chain, which meant that Mary would need to approach Chief Maxson before mentioning the leggings nonsense to any other superior officer.

But this was a problematic proposition, given Mary's brief history with Chief Maxson. She'd already received multiple demerits. In fact, there'd been so many that Mary had begun to refer to Maxson as "Chiefee" behind her back.

Mary could muster courage if her friends asked it of her, so she promised to ask the colonel if Chief Maxson said no. As predicted, Chief Maxson decreed that the leggings were army-issue and, therefore, the nurses would wear them as ordered. But the next day Mary saw Col. Bracher briefly and mentioned the leggings issue. He said that her assertion made complete sense to him and ordered that each nurse should save their leggings until cold weather necessitated their use.

Despite the great news regarding the leggings and the arrival of such a wonderful nurse as Alabama, Lorraine's chuckle and good-natured demeanor had all but disappeared. Her negative attitude toward virtually every task required in maneuvers training morphed to lamentation and then outright depression. September was even worse than August. It was still blistering hot during the day, but autumn's night chills froze their damp skin. She and Mary had resorted to sleeping on one cot together just to try to stay warm.

By mid-September, Lorraine's ankle pain worsened. It had not been given the chance to heal properly because of the physical hardships they all endured that summer. In fact, when Mary could grab a few minutes to help her ice it and Lorraine felt relief from the ankle pain, she realized that all the other joints in her body ached. She wasn't sure why, but she decided not to confess to Mary that she was hurting everywhere. Something was wrong, though. She was a nurse, after all. She began experiencing a premonition that there was more than a decent chance that she would be physically unable to endure maneuvers once summer fully succumbed to autumn. But Mary and Mona, among others, misinterpreted Lorraine's disdain for maneuvers, chalking it up to a poor attitude that she was well within her reach to change.[1]

All the nurses' morale is low but believe Lorraine's is the worst. She absolutely refuses to adjust and gripes worse than I do. The trouble is she spouts off at the wrong time and her attitude reflects upon me as we are together so much. The chief has been giving us opposite hours and today she blew her top about that. Personally, I don't care as I think we see enough of each other as is. Tonite Mona and I had a little chat and Mona being the sweetest, most generous friend a girl could have, … and also being a little older and much wiser than myself said she wished we could do things together more often like go to Nashville, etc… She said that we'll probably be happier because we won't demand as much. She has some wonderful philosophy and a heart-to-heart talk with her does me a world of good. No, we

---

1   Later in life, Lorraine was diagnosed with arthritis. She was possibly symptomatic as early as 1943.

don't like this any better than Lorraine does, but as far as I can see there's no sense in raving about it from dawn till dark. She hates calisthenics, drill, hikes, etc. Well, I'm glad I went in for those things in high school as they don't bother me a bit and I really think we need the calisthenics as much as we sit around on duty.

Despite not feeling well, Lorraine forced herself to accompany Mary to the Hotel Dixie in Shelbyville, Tennessee. It was known for the best fried chicken in town, and shops were within walking distance.

I purchased a pair of woolen khaki socks, some bubble earrings to match my necklace and bracelet (don't ask me when I'm going to have the opportunity to wear them), some tomatoes and peaches, a little carbide lamp, you'd laugh if you saw it, also a little stove which burns canned heat—this for hot water to wash my face, as this darn old cold creek water is so hard on my complexion.

After finishing our shopping, the hostess at the Hotel Dixie was determined to see that Lorraine and I had a wonderful meal. Real Southern fried chicken, each a half one, tossed salad, the nearest to yours, Mom, that I've had since leaving home, French fries, toasted buns, iced tea and ice cream. These Southerners really treat us very graciously and are so interested in our lives and work. But such junky towns I've never seen—dirty and dilapidated and ancient. The women wear sunbonnets, and it is a common site to see horse and buggy. They even sell them.

Got into a little Dutch later because after our wonderful dinner we were about to head back to camp and ran into four Air Corps officers. They asked us to go someplace and dance. We didn't see what we had to lose so they ushered us to a civilian car, and we rode about five miles from the town and stopped at some club where we drank cokes and danced. Then we headed back to Shelbyville for a late sandwich. All of the sudden as we were eating the sirens sounded, and boom, we were caught in a blackout. The officers had to be signed in by 11:30 p.m., and we had to get back, too, praying that Chiefee would be sleeping during blackout conditions and not know that we were still out on the town. Of course, no such luck. Next morning, we were informed by "her highness" that Lorraine and I would be separated not only with opposing shifts but recreational activities as well. No more nights out together…

The separation became permanent. On October 2, 1943, Chief Maxson ordered Lorraine to be transferred to Camp Gordon, a station hospital in Georgia. Mary agonized over her departure. It would be more than two years before they would see each other again.

If I had known, I would have tried to help Lorraine out by washing her navy slacks and then getting a corpsman to iron them. (We are not allowed to iron. Not sure why.) It all started because last night Lorraine wore brown slacks instead of the required navy ones. She tried to explain to Chief that the laundry can't do navy slacks, and she thought that she had made the correct decision to wear the clean brown ones because her navy ones were filthy. But this morning there was a little typewritten notice on the tree in front of her majesty's tent that said:

"No sloppiness of army nurses will be tolerated in the field any more than in garrison. GI shoes will be worn at all times. Improper wearing of insignia will not be tolerated. Coverall legs will not be rolled, etc.

The army expects RESULTS—NOT EXCUSES."

CHAPTER 9

Pickled Caterpillars and Wood Tick Juice

Mona had a way with Chief Maxson that bore similarities to Mary's way with Col. Bracher. Once Lorraine vacated their most recent cow pasture and the girls' tent, Mona asked Chief Maxson if Alabama could move in with her and Mary. Alabama would prove to be a faithful, dependable friend to the other tent mates for the duration of her service in the 39th.

October 8, 1943
Dear Family:
    Am writing this on duty and trying to think of an excuse to not go to the Country Club for an officers' party tonight. I'm in no mood to go since Chiefee finally succeeded in separating Lorraine and me. I wish it could have been me that she sent away, as I think that I could adjust to a new environment better. I feel as if I've lost my right arm or something.
    Oh, you would get the biggest kick out of the ward boys. They've been so cute—all coming around to my wards singing "Mary's a Grand Ole Name" and offering their sympathies because my buddy and I were separated. They're all asking if they can take Lorraine's place now.
    I went by myself to Nashville to forget my troubles. I did a little shopping, met some paratroopers, went to the Hermitage for dinner, and danced to a lovely orchestra. Then I made my way to the "High Hat" and danced with practically every private, corporal, etc., in the place. In fact, I struggled to get off the floor. Guess the civilian girls envied me, but I was envying them in their pretty clothes. All the soldiers told me that I was too young to be a lieutenant and not the type for the army. And here I thought that I had already acquired that hard GI appearance.
    Got back to camp about 1:30 a.m., and guess who was waiting up for me? Mona. She had my bed all fixed and made a fire as she had surmised that I would be so cold after having ridden the two hours from Nashville in an open truck. She also thought how dreadful it was going to be to come back to our tent and know that Lorraine wouldn't be here. Felt lousy this morning so didn't get up for calisthenics or chow, so Alabama came back from chow with their mess kits full of a nice hot breakfast for me…

During October, Mona made a conscious decision to not take the time necessary for keeping track of Mary's belongings. In fact, like Inga and Nancy before her, she recognized that Mary was more than capable of the self-motivation necessary for taking on the trivialities inherent in everyday existence. As long as Lorraine had been present (continually for the past year and a half), Mary remained juvenile. Almost out of some bizarre unsaid pact between her and her childhood friend, Lorraine organized Mary's life (e.g., sewing, packing) and, in turn, Mary psychologically supported Lorraine by reflecting her negative attitude toward virtually every activity associated with maneuvers training.

With Lorraine gone, her friends cared for Mary in more overt ways (such as bringing her breakfast or fixing her bed) only because she would do the same for them if they came in late from town. But the covert coddling ceased the minute Lorraine boarded the two-ton for Georgia on that fall day in Tennessee.

Although Lorraine and Mary probably scored equally regarding the number of times each had been disciplined, Mona surmised that perhaps there had been a discussion among their superiors (Col. Bracher, Major Scanlon, Lt. Maxson) to determine which nurse to remove from Tennessee maneuvers. Mary was a steady, talented bedside nurse with a nose for diagnostics, but Lorraine had been heralded as a fine surgical nurse. Of course, Lorraine's health had deteriorated in Tennessee. Surely that had been a factor contributing to her exit. And, if they were bound for Europe, maybe choosing Mary to remain in the unit had to do with Mary being fluent in German. Mary would be called on to translate. It could be that German prisoners of war might comprise a portion of their patient load over there.

They often wondered if fate or God had played a part, but in the end, they decided the "why" was irrelevant. The army's superiors made decisions regarding the "who," the "when," the "where," and most assuredly, the "why." By fall 1943, both Mary and Mona understood that, as soldiers very low on the decision-making pole, they were only responsible for carrying out the "what."

October 17, 1943

Colonel Scott, a full Colonel, has been with us for 3 days. He returned from the Theatre of Operations (in Italy) a week ago and talked to us for 2 hrs. Thurs. He is the CO of the first Evacuation Hospital to be set up in this war. They took part in the Tunisian Campaign and also in the Sicilian battles. He told us exactly how an evacuation hospital operates in combat. It is directly behind the front lines. The medical unit has nurses that close to the front. He told us how fortunate that we were to be with an evac. hosp. in this war as it's really this unit that gets the first casualties. They moved at least every ten days, half the time on foot. They cared for all casualties—American, German, French. He also said that the Germans have respected all hospitals over there unless it was purely accidental. Out of 2700 casualties receiving aid in ten days at their hospital only thirteen of them died as he traced those cases back. Of course, many of them are in Africa in general hospital, but all are expected to recover fully.

He told us the facts, no glamour attached, how important discipline of every member of the group is and must be. He lauded his nurses and the whole ANC and told Chiefee that a sleeping bag was a "must have" as most of the time they sleep on the ground.

We are to be instructed in the giving of blood transfusions and plasma. Plasma is the main life saver, and they have the plasma bottles marked "colored" for the colored boys.[1] They use morphine to avert shock, which formerly was the main killer. Soldiers are issued morphine syrettes before going into battle, but they load the evac. hospitals with it, too, once patients arrive from the battlefields. Officers are also given Benzedrine. In Tunisia, he said they had to deal with lots of broken bones, especially ankles.

Colonel Scott said that his evac. hospital lived on C Rations for five months and are all still healthy. Of course, they took vitamins and a lot of concentrated stuff. He doesn't know exactly when we will go, but he assures us that we will and that our group of nurses here will definitely go with the 39th. We will be given twenty more nurses at POE (Point of Embarkation.)

P. S. Have you ever tried pickled caterpillars with wood tick juice—or coffee-flavored flies for dessert? That's what one of the soldiers asked me last night on our way back to camp.

Nov. 22, 1943
Dearest Daddy:

A few lines to post you on latest developments in the 39th. I've had a feeling that things would start happening around here as we've been out in the field training longer than any other evacuation hospital. Today we received the news that we are alerted.[2]

Zim and I had beautiful plans for Christmas, but once more they have crumbled. Guess everything nice must wait until after the war. From now on, if my letters seem less than forthcoming you understand that it's because of potential censoring. Chiefee warned us this morning that we must be careful from now on.

I thought that if I wrote to you, Daddy, you could break the news to Mom a little easier. Tomorrow, we get our teeth checked. We also have to make out a will.

It's so cold here tonight, Daddy, and I'm so thankful for the sleeping bag you bought me...

December 6, 1943
Dearest Family,

Gosh, it's been a while since I wrote. Chiefee's been on the warpath lately and really laid me out about my financial troubles. (Nothing gets by her and she thinks that my finances are indicative of my anti-soldier tendencies.) Guess I'm her problem child. She must not worry about me as a nurse, though. She now has assigned three wards to me, and boy they sure keep me hopping.

All us girls are so disgusted around here. We were alerted many days ago and still we sit. Anyway, it was our five-month anniversary in the field, and we are all sick to death of it. If we have to go to war, we're all saying to get over there already. Think we've got the hang of maneuvers by now, for goodness sakes...

---

1   The practice of differentiating blood based on race was very offensive to Mary. During World War II, a U.S. Army standard protocol was that the bottles of blood plasma donated by a person of color should be marked "colored." Mary's letter becomes a foreshadowing of an experience she would have during the Battle of the Bulge.

2   This meant that a unit had been put on notice that it would be going overseas to war.

December 10, 1943
Dear Family,

Today we all rode in a 6 × 6 to Camp Forrest to have our eyes examined. Had a very thorough exam and was relieved to find out that I don't need GI glasses. On the way back to camp it was raining pitchforks and the canvas covering the old truck leaked something awful, but we sang the entire 20 miles back and kept up the ole GI spirit. We envied the nurses we saw in their white uniforms, but I like my outfit so well and am so used to outdoor life by now believe I'm just as happy here. I would hate to go back to civilian life now and hope I don't ever have to until after this war. The ANC means a great deal to me. And golly I've made so many wonderful friends—well—they just couldn't be any better. Mona is so darn sweet and without her doubt if I could survive some of our trying days.

Corporal Davis got my small radio to working just perfectly, but there's not enough power in our area for the large one so am going to rent it to one of the boys who has a wife in town. I know he'll take excellent care of it, and I'll be making a profit which I'll send to you if you'd like, especially since I'm always in debt to my family, including my sisters.

Have been wrapping some gifts for the boys, mailing their packages in town, and sewing on stripes and more stripes—it all helps to keep me occupied, and I enjoy doing things for them…

December 17, 1943
Dearest Mom and Dad,

Here I sit on a real bed with a real mattress. Mona is fixing her nails. We are having an overnight at the Hotel Dixie in Shelbyville as tomorrow we have a day off to do our Christmas shopping. Have been so sick with the flu and so busy since our orders came. We are to move on Monday, back to garrison, Camp Forrest, TN, twenty miles from Shelbyville. Of course, everyone is very happy at the prospect, but we won't be working in the hospital. The 39th will be in an area all our own—all of our nurses in one barracks. Our days will consist of six to eight hours of classes, going on long hikes and learning to drive GI vehicles. Chiefee says that we'll be there for about six weeks for this phase of our training.

Mona and I are so glad to get into a hotel bed even for just one night as Wednesday we had to move out in the field again. They didn't put our living tents up since we'll just be there a few days, though, so they have all twenty of us nurses in one big ward tent—barely enough room to move around, no place to hang our clothes and colder than blazes. This morning there was ice on the tent walls, the water in the water trailers was frozen solid, and the water in my canteen cup which I had placed under my bunk before going to sleep was a solid mass of ice when I woke up. Everyone is taking the conditions with a grin and morale is good in spite of it all. It just doesn't seem real that our maneuver life is almost over. Just so happy that I get to go overseas with this outfit, the truest and best friends in the world, and if and when we have to face this war so glad that we have each other. Once we're over there suppose we will laugh at the simple hardships we endured in Tennessee.

Mona and I came into town around six p.m. I had my hair fixed and then six of us came up to Mona's and my room, took baths, ate, and fooled around until dinner. I'm so tired because I was on night duty last night so slept in my frozen bunk only two hours. While on duty, everybody razzed me—the doctors were mad because the boys didn't stay on their wards but spent all their time talking to me, the patients complained that it sounded like Grand Central Station, but I was enjoying it in spite of feeling rotten.

Haven't heard from Zim and know he's angry that I'm going overseas. Well, why should he wait for me? Know I won't be the same girl when I come back, but I signed up with Uncle Sam for the duration and intend to do my best for our boys. My reward is their appreciation. I'll probably end up a hard old spinster, but even if I do, my life and these girls who are serving with me will have been fuller than lots of others I know.

Next week we are to have a vacation—to prepare us for what's coming, I guess…

December 20 marked the final day for what had been a grueling five months of maneuvers training in middle Tennessee. The 39th received orders to pack up and move to Camp Forrest (named after confederate Nathan Bedford Forrest) in Tullahoma, Tennessee. The 39th joined other troops stationed there, but the evac occupied a separate part of the camp. Beginning on December 21, Mary was held to an even more restricted space at their new digs, a result of another lack of judgment on her part.

Dear Family,

Good grief—here I sit in Brownie's room. (Brownie's one of our only married nurses and a wonderful person.) She's letting me borrow her radio while I write letters and keep up with my diary since the vacation I was due is now completely ruined. At noon today I got doled out a seven-day restriction from the old battleax. Everybody, even Mona this time, feels sorry for me because of the latest mess I've gotten myself into. But this one seems innocent to everybody in the 39th, except for the one who counts—Chiefee.

And the guy who should carry the blame is on maneuvers for at least three weeks so no help from any testimony he may have offered on my behalf, the wolf. He's really not a wolf, and very handsome. He was in the movie "Silver Skates," went to Law College, rich so he has his own car here and that's why the trouble started. Had a date with him last night and, of course, I was more impressed with the car than anything else he had to offer. Guess I made too much of a big deal about his having the darn Buick and he offered to let me have it for the weeks he's on maneuvers, even giving me tons of gas coupons to tear around on. So I was on the beam after our date, dreaming up various plans for taking the girls around during our vacation week, thinking about shopping opportunities, Christmas purchases I could make for my patients who can't get out of the hospital to shop for their moms and girlfriends, etc.

Well, everything in my head was lovely and on the way back from taking Bill to his quarters (about six miles away from our quarters) the darn car stopped. I tried everything to get it to crank but to no avail, so I found a guard who in turn found a fellow to take me back to my quarters. I ran into Mona and her lieutenant that she dated last night, and he offered to go see about the car. I told him that it might just be out of gas, but later he called and said he got it to crank and that he decided that he better drive it to a garage in town to have a mechanic look at it to make sure nothing major is wrong. So now I can't go get the car for the entire time it would have been helpful to have it in the first place because by the time I get off restriction my vacation will be over.

So, the reason I'm on restriction is because I stepped in mud in my good shoes when I tried to find someone to help me with the stalled car. I didn't have time to clean the shoes because I didn't get back to quarters until 4 a.m. and slept until 11:30 when Mona came and woke me and said we had class beginning at noon. I barely had time to find anything that I was supposed to wear. I put on some toeless black play shoes that I knew were not right, but I didn't dare miss class. Then I began looking for my overseas cap but remembered that I had left it in Lt. Emerson's car last night so the only cap I had was my garrison cap. Anyway, I figured that if I missed class that would be a bigger problem than showing up out of uniform, so I decided on the latter and, at least, after class I got to eat dinner before my punishment went into full force. Chiefee said that it will last seven days, and she will allow me to go to meals and our own PX, absolutely no shopping in town, and no Christmas parties. There's to be a party for all officers in the Officers' Day Room on Christmas Day, but she won't let me attend. It stinks—but definitely.

So, a few hours ago Ms. Battleax found me holed up in Brownie's room and said, "Lt. Balster, I need you to help decorate the nurses' Christmas tree since you have plenty of time on your hands."

I followed Chiefee to the parlor and actually enjoyed helping her decorate. I suppose she wants me to sit in my room and mope for seven days but darned if I'll give her the satisfaction. I said, "Chief Maxson, do you mind if I bring Brownie's radio out here to the parlor and we can listen to Christmas music while we decorate? My daddy always had the radio on back home when he would do our tree, or he asked my sister Nancy to play carols on the piano and we sang. Nancy also plays the organ just like you. I really do love to hear you play the organ at church. You are such a gifted musician."

Chiefee is good on the organ, and I really didn't mean to sound disingenuous, but I think she did not take the compliment very well because she said that we could do without the radio and wouldn't be that long decorating such a small tree. I said, "Yes ma'am."

(Three hours later) Well, Chiefee was right—it took less than an hour to do the tree and then I told Chiefee that if there was nothing else that she needed I really should wash out all of my muddy clothes. It's so nice to have access to hot water after five months in the field, but, of course, about an hour ago she put her nose in it and said, "Lt. Balster, you're using far too much hot water for your fatigues." I replied, "Yes ma'am," and went on washing with the hot water—even my housecoat needed it, as it was worse than any of my army clothes.

Despite the seven-day restriction, Chief Maxson allowed Mary to walk the 2 miles to the mess hall to get a great Christmas meal—fruit, candy, nuts, turkey with all the trimmings, hot biscuits, and mincemeat pie, all thanks to Leon, the chef from Milwaukee.

Restriction wasn't all bad. After all, she had time to jot down memories of the difficult summer and fall. As for the spring, all recollections centered around Zim. At night, she held the little castle insignia he'd given her. It represented his role as engineer in the service. Her stomach tightened and her hands tingled every time she eyed a castle insignia on someone's uniform. But she couldn't allow herself to fall into daydreams about marrying him. The likelihood of that prospect at this point in her life was so minuscule that to create such fantasies in her mind would hurt too much. She was about to go to war, for goodness' sakes. Too, there was another sobering fact—while the content of Zim's letters was lengthy, there were very few of them. Or was she being inconsiderate? He was very busy, in charge of the 1,000-yard rifle range.

Also, there was the distinct possibility that his being male may have something to do with his lackluster letter volume. But still, there were too many strikes against a future with him. She had made a commitment to Uncle Sam, and she intended to keep it.

After Mary had served out her restriction, her Christmas packages from family had arrived, so she opened them in Camp Forrest's Recreation Hall. Her best officer friends looked on in celebration of her release. She and Mona recalled the time that Mary had opened all those lost packages and boxes in front of Zim. It seemed a lifetime ago, not a mere seven months.

This time, ingenious Inga had wrapped all the Swedish cookies in unsalted popcorn as a method for keeping the fragile cookies fresh and unbroken. Even though small white pellets of popcorn stuck to the jelly-filled cookies, the guys and gals picked off the popcorn remnants and commented how the cookies tasted as if Inga had baked them that very day.

> All the boys say they're following me home to St. Paul when this darn war is over. They said they just can't decide if they'll go first to Daddy's restaurant or to my house because everything I get sent from either place is divine. I told them that my family would love every one of them and would treat them like kings, which they all are.

Mary watched her Ps and Qs around Chief Maxson so as not to miss the midnight fireworks slated for New Year's Eve. And she'd go stag, as that was the most efficient way to ensure her sticking to the rules. She may have been her own worst enemy, but to add a man to the mix certainly never helped. She'd learned that much and stuck to a life free from love for a little over a month.

> January 3, 1944
> Dearest Mom and Dad,
>
> Am waiting for Lt. Emerson to call from Nashville again. Have to try to make arrangements for him to get his darn car back. This has been a fiasco. Ever since the car got out of the shop different guys have been borrowing it, using all the gas coupons, and I'm a nervous wreck that one of them is going to crash it and then what the heck am I supposed to do? Of course, it's a big joke around the post and I'm forever being teased about it.
>
> (Later that same evening) We had to sit in the parlor and wait in line to be measured for our OD (Olive Drab). I was sure hoping that I'd hear the phone ring and they'd yell "Mary, a Lt. Emerson is on the line," but he never called. Regarding the uniforms, we will be issued two suits, shirts, capes, trench coats, shoes, a bag, gloves, seersucker dresses, overcoats, etc. Where they are taking us is still a secret. Maybe they don't even know yet but guess they expect it to be somewhere cold. Gad, I have enough shoes now to start a factory. Today I bought an OD comforter for $2.98 and was able to sell my mattress for $2.00! They made me buy a scout knife, some OD bath towels and said that we needed to buy soap and toothpaste every time we go to the PX to start stocking up. Everything from underwear out has to be OD.

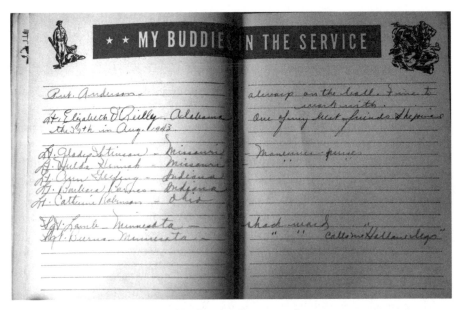

Mary lists friends in her service diary

Mona laid out her equipment on her bunk. Chief Maxson was due any moment for inspection. Tent pegs, ropes, gas mask, helmet, etc. Yes, all accounted for.

Mary looked over at Mona's army issued equipment. In comparison, hers wasn't going to pass muster. She was missing several tent pegs and ropes. She had no idea where the anti-dim for the gas mask was. And her helmet's straps were burned off. The iron had fallen directly on the straps when she'd gone to check on a patient. Maxson decided to forego asking Mary why she was ironing on duty in the first place since the rules specifically stated that nurses weren't allowed to iron.

But all she said was, "Well, I'd say that you're just about *half here*, aren't you Lt.?"

***

The 39th spent approximately six weeks at Camp Forrest before making way to Camp Kilmer, New Jersey, a training installation designed to prepare troops for overseas. Camp Kilmer was massive, housing over 1.3 million soldiers who were either waiting for deployment or awaiting new training assignments.

The camp boasted 20 softball diamonds and 30 volleyball courts and had its own band and orchestra.[3] Everyone appreciated the food. Fresh fruit was delivered every morning to their room.

Dagny Solberg, another nurse in the 39th, had a penchant for army life. She was a great soldier but also enjoyed traveling and loved New York. Mary and Mona had seen Dagny work countless hours while they were training, as if she had no regard for any physical ailment she may have been suffering. Her determination and will for service were top priority, but she knew how to enjoy life, too. She had been sick with a cold, but Mary knew a "little sniffle" wouldn't deter Dagny. And a head cold wouldn't dissuade Mary from having a day in New York, either.

Mary and Mona had opted out of paying for maid service while at Camp Kilmer and instead decided to divvy up the cleaning tasks and save that $5.50 each toward a nice meal in the city. Mona arranged for transportation into New York while Mary made ready for a new chance at inspection. With Mona's help, she passed that one.

Mary coughed so much on the George Washington Bridge that Mona and Dagny decided a very stiff Tom Collins at the Biltmore Lounge must take precedence over shopping at Lord and Taylor. While she appreciated their concern, her consumption of hard liquor had been expended in Tullahoma when she was so inebriated that for a week afterwards, she'd endured incessant teasing and ribbing by other officers. She'd be sticking to champagne or wine from now on. Her favorite ward boy Poncho would be receiving all her future liquor rations.

At the Waldorf, they dined on shrimp cocktail, fresh brook trout, cauliflower, potatoes, rolls, salad, rum raisin ice cream, wafers, and coffee. The meal totaled $3.95. Mona recalled that they'd paid only $2.50 for steak and fries recently, but that was in the South.

After dinner, they took the guided tour through Rockefeller Center, including Radio City, and saw the city by night from the Observation Tower. Breathtaking, they said. Then they went to the Crossroads for coffee and sardine sandwiches.

Mary's only regret was that her taste was on the blink from her cold, so some of that good food went to waste. But everyone was suffering with colds and nasty coughs. Who could complain? It was New York.

---

3   Camp Kilmer was the largest processing center for troops going overseas and returning from the European Theater of Operations during World War II.

Wish you could see Mona and me right now. We are wearing our brown and white seersucker dresses surrounded by papers and letters littering our bunks with just enough leftover room to sit. Mona's writing to her boyfriend and is wasting a lot of paper as she's tearing the letters up as fast as she writes and now is asking *me* for ideas. Gad, I have a hard enough time on my own. I've not heard from Zim in over a month. Not sure if his letters can't catch up with me, or if he's gotten word that I've given up hope for any future with him. Every time I see a castle insignia my heart sinks. No matter how many shave tails to Lt. Colonels I've dated since Zim, I know that I am still smitten with him. A certain song or a smell or a dance has the power to instantly send me back to Ft. Wood. I hope that he feels the same about me when certain life moments jolt his memories.

And my love life isn't my only concern. Once again, my finances are worrying me. How much did my luggage cost? I paid three mess bills in one month that amounted to $50.00. I think that I can scrape up enough to pay you back for the luggage, but I'd prefer to wait until the overseas allotments start coming my way, but that should be very soon, I believe…

PART II

HMS *Andes* and Altrincham
Spring 1944–Summer 1944

CHAPTER 10

Shave Tail

On a pier at the Port of New York, the Red Cross served coffee and donuts while a band played "The Victory March." Although the pageantry was small, the collective mood of the 39th was anything but subdued. Earned pride felt different than the superficial pride that Mary had felt the first night at Fort Leonard Wood. She could see that now. She deserved to be walking the gangplank to board the HMS *Andes*. Three months of nursing at Wood; five months of grueling maneuvers training in god-awful Tennessee; around 60 romantic evenings with Zim and then being forced to say goodbye to him, possibly forever; a lifetime with Lorraine and then the awful separation from her, also possibly forever; the boys she'd cared for, the one with the ruptured appendix whom she saved from dying—all of these experiences, they made her feel deserving to march on this gangplank for parts unknown. No idea where they were going. No idea how long they would be there. Not one glimpse into the future. All she knew was that at this moment she deserved to be where she was. She deserved to serve. And she had a funny feeling that everyone who marched in front of her and behind her felt the same.

During the first couple of days in February 1944, Col. Bracher focused his efforts on compiling the final list of personnel who would sail for service overseas. Some received last-minute transfers during the unit's stint at Camp Kilmer. A few were deemed too ill for service out of country. But the majority of the 39th's officers and enlisted personnel who'd trained at Camp Atterbury, at Fort Leonard Wood, and who had completed maneuvers training in Tennessee boarded the HMS *Andes* on February 8, 1944. As to where they were headed, latrine rumors were rampant. Some said Africa. The only certainty that Chief Maxson offered her 48 female nurses was that they would run a hospital while on board to support the 2,000 male soldiers from the 203rd Anti-Aircraft Artillery Automatic Weapons Battalion, the 635th Tank Destroyer Battalion, and the 1195th Engineer Combat Group.[1] Some would probably get seasick. Still others would need immunizations like typhoid shots. And statistics dictated that out of 2,000 men, there would be the usual mix of pneumonia, flu, formerly undiagnosed malaria and the like.

Once the tugboats pulled the *Andes* into the open waters of the Atlantic, it was safe to announce their destination. They were headed to the British Isles and would be docking in Liverpool, hopefully in 10 days or less. Blackout conditions were to be observed at all times. No lights would be allowed on the main deck and all windows from which light might show were going to be covered with black cloths.

Chief Maxson announced that her nurses would be allowed the rest of the day off to unpack and tour the hospital. A schedule would be posted at the nurses' station the following day at 0500. This was not a pleasure cruise, but in the minds of the nurses, it certainly felt like one already, especially when one considered that the men outnumbered the women 45 to one.

Mona and Mary would share a small cabin, but they were told they'd been lucky to have been assigned a stateroom at all. Mona took on the sole task of locating their domicile. Mary had gone to daydreaming already, her mind in a swirl of delight, consumed with pleasing images of a handsome second lieutenant they'd met during the briefing.

She asked Mona if she'd noticed his eyes. Mona didn't answer. She was concentrating on the map of the ship.

Biggest brown irises Mary had ever seen, but definitely. Eyelashes any gal would envy. He was one of those men who had the potential to get even better-looking 10 years down the road when some of the roundness of that baby face wore off for good… looked to be about the same age as Zim, 25 maybe? Did Mona recall how tall he was? Mary couldn't remember. Who cared anyway? Golly, those eyes. He was a southerner. Yes, she'd sworn off dating any more southern men. But his accent sounded like Alabama's. It had a refinement to it; didn't Mona think so?

Mona breathed an "aha," as she finally found the tiny stateroom. Did Mary recall that it wasn't just southern men she'd sworn off? She thought that going stag was now the rule of thumb because Mary's commitment to Uncle Sam was above all else. Or had she forgotten that?

She hadn't, but this day had turned out so wonderfully. After all, the weather was stunning. The sea sparkled. The good will and God-speed wishes from

1   HMS *Andes*, WW2troopships.com & WWIItrooopships.com, Web Site Copyright 2007 Shayne E. Wallesch & Wendy J. Hochnadel.

the Red Cross personnel. How wonderful was that? The feeling of patriotism. The pride. The men, so many of them. And then that southern shave tail to boot.[2] Only the dead could remain unenthused, for goodness' sakes.

Besides, she was also committed to other acts of self-improvement, one being to not assume that all southerners were dumb as bricks. Alabama bore testament to that, so Mary was making strides not to immediately stereotype when she heard a southern accent.

Mona didn't want to bring up a sore subject, but Chief Maxson had been pleased with Mary's non-dating policy of late. If Mary was planning to pursue finding that southerner again, it would be difficult to hide him. After all, 48 nurses and their behaviors would easily be noticeable on a ship with 2,000 men.

Mary wasn't concerned about Chiefee. Her only concern was the 2,000 men part. How would she ever be able to find that lieutenant again? If she did, the best option where Chiefee was concerned would be to just avoid her as much as humanly possible. Knowing her, she'd probably spend most of her time down in the hospital anyway. Mary would only have to see her during shift assignments. Besides, the fresh sea air had reminded Mary of just how big the world was. Chiefee's world was so small. She'd figured out Chiefee's problem. Chiefee was just hopelessly middle class. In the real world, Chiefee was a non-entity. Perspective was a grand and glorious thing to own.

But this Lt. Roberson, this gentleman, now he was a man to be examined further. What a face. Didn't even matter that his haircut was a mess. "What I mean!"[3] she muttered as Mona asked if Mary wouldn't mind taking the top bunk.

Never mind about the top bunk. It was fine. Her primary concern centered on finding the southern shave tail, especially with blackout conditions being enforced. Did she hear correctly that he said he'd be on the lookout for her?

She didn't have cause for worry. Robby found her just prior to sunset. She was easy to spot, the only one on deck who scurried about like a lost goose on the way to chow.

February 12, 1944
Dearest Family,
 The ocean is beautiful today, the white caps positively glisten. Am sitting on my upper bunk watching the waves go by. So far have really been enjoying this trip and (along with only a few others) hold the record for not getting a bit seasick, but better I should keep my fingers crossed.

---

2 "Shave tail" was Army slang for second lieutenant.
3 "What I mean" was 1940s slang equivalent to millennial slang for, "Damn, he's hot."

Yesterday worked in the ship's hospital (we take turns). We wear our brown and white seersucker dresses with those cute little caps to match. It was so much fun doing some nursing for a change.

We are very comfortable, the food is excellent, and my new boyfriend divine. He is a rebel—cute and fun to be with. Met him on deck our first day on ship. Last night we went to the entertainment, and this morning we watched the ocean together, and in a little while we are meeting in the lounge to spend the afternoon together.

He's a shave tail by the way...

Notwithstanding a couple of day shifts, Mary spent every waking hour with the shave tail nicknamed Robby. As it turned out, Chief Maxson spent most of the voyage holed up with seasickness, thus unable to track Mary's whereabouts. In fact, many on the ship were sick, caused by the captain's decision to alter the *Andes'* original route and head toward rough seas. Even though the threat of German U-boats was almost non-existent by early 1944, there'd been chatter that some sort of enemy threat had been spotted. The ship was outfitted with decent artillery, but the *Andes* didn't have a military escort for this voyage, so the captain altered the original route and turned her due north. For the next several days, seas slapped and tossed about her 25,689 gross tonnage like a plastic toy boat in a bathtub.

To Mary's great fortune, she and her new-found love continued to be unaffected by the head seas.

... Yesterday morning, I worked in the hospital again and fell down twice, my dinner slid right out from under my nose, and I came back to our stateroom and fell in the bathtub and still am not any the worse for wear. The sea is a bit rough, and we haven't been allowed outside for a couple of days.

We were told that this voyage was not a pleasure cruise but to me it has been... Had a Valentine party—the officers gave each of us a cute valentine with an original verse on each one...

I've learned to play Blackjack and won $1.00 the first time I played, but I lost it last night. We just play with nickels. Everyone laughs at me the way I play cards, but we have fun anyway, even though there's no liquor allowed on this ship.

You know, when a man tells you he loves you when he hasn't been drinking it seems to mean a little more than when he has. Of course, they all tell the gals that anyway—guess that's just part of their GI line, but with this one I'm using my own lines now too so guess we're even... My gosh, Daddy, I think I'm in love again, and don't laugh.

Will end this now, as it's time for my friend to appear again. He stands outside our door and sings "Mary is a Grand Ole Name" in his rebel brogue...

Naturally, Robby was partial to southern food, always salted with "fat back," so the bland British food on the ship was a disappointment. Sardines were the saltiest things he could get his hands on, so he stuck to those. Alcohol wasn't permitted on the *Andes*. In lieu of it, he and Mary drank fruit juice and shared multiple cans of peaches.

Robby never met a stranger. The lieutenants in his unit called out to him constantly, "Robby, who's that you got wich ya?" "Oh, this is my little ole Yankee gal, Mary." They were overjoyed that Robby had found love.

Alabama and Robby were instant friends. She said he was the kind of young man that everybody wanted the best for—his subordinates and superiors alike. Of course, the women liked him. What gal wouldn't? His eyes, in color and shape, looked like southern pecans that had been glazed with melted butter. She wondered if Mary ever compared him to Zim. Even though Alabama hadn't met Zim, she'd certainly been privy to Mary's pining over his absence during maneuvers.

His smile was like Zim's except that Robby's had that endearing small gap in the two front teeth. Zim was a bit conceited. Robby, never. He wasn't the least bit vain about his superior looks. There was strut in his gait, yes, but no false pride connected with it, no moxie at all. Just sheer joy to be alive. Everyone gravitated to Zim because he was a natural-born leader. With Robby, people were drawn to him because of his manner, his infectious zeal for living each moment. And his eyes had a look of reassurance, especially when he knew that she was anxious. He was like Zim in that way, except that he was far more positive. Zim was cynical, not just about the war but about life in general. But Robby, no. There was nothing more to him than good looks, pragmatism, honesty, generosity of spirit, and passionate optimism. What more could a gal want?

Alabama wholeheartedly agreed.

It became habit for Robby to stroll with Mary on deck in the late evening and eventually escort her to the cabin she shared with Mona. She kept her hopes up that Robby would offer more affection than just the kiss on her hand, but she decided that his ability to resist her had a connection to that darned moral code that seemed to define him. She was conflicted. On the one hand, she felt honored that Robby held himself to such discipline that he would not dare kiss her on the mouth so soon into their courtship. On the other hand, she dreamed of the night that he would advance his affections just a bit.

Later, Robby commented that by about the fourth or fifth day on the HMS *Andes*, he had begun to acknowledge to himself that he felt an emptiness in his gut about this gal. It really didn't matter what she did or how she handled herself in whatever circumstance. He was certain that he was smitten. She was an absolute pleasure, her beauty so boldly feminine, her approach to life so naïve. But there was that hidden grit about her that absolutely mystified him.

Why she always sought to cover up that sheer will of hers with that flighty, goofy persona he didn't know. She had so much substance, but she always insisted on pretending that she had none. It was an intriguing act, though. He'd never known any gal like her.

By the seventh day of the voyage, the two already were discussing marriage. They both adored children, and during their strolls, they promised each other that they would start working on having "six little Rebels" as soon as the war was behind them. And Robby said somehow, he would find an opportunity to get an engagement ring and propose properly. If he couldn't, he would send money to one of his sisters to shop for a ring stateside.

When Robby asked Mary what her mother would think about their talks of marriage, especially since they'd known each other for less than two weeks, she speculated that at first it would cause Inga's head to swirl, but then she'd probably chalk it up to another of Mary's impulsivities. And as far as her father went, whatever Mary did was golden, other than her decision to join the service behind his back.

The more he learned about Mary's sheltered upbringing, he wondered how she'd developed that strength that she was forever trying to hide. Aside from the maneuvers in Tennessee, it didn't seem as if Mary had ever known misery. He had grown up with it.

The Depression had left him and his family hungry for years. He felt so used up by the time the 1930s were over that the only feeling in him stronger than his sense of patriotism was his sense that the U.S. entering the world's war might offer him an opportunity to help his family financially. He joined the National Guard in Greenwood, Mississippi, as soon as he'd finished his obligation with the WPA's work on building the Enid Dam, just north of Charleston, Mississippi, where he had grown up in a family of nine children.

Robby's Guard training had begun at Camp Blanding, Florida, but soon after enlisting and proving to own smarts and leadership skills, he was recommended for Officers' Training School. In Mary's service diary, she penned a dash next to his name with the words "the only GI I ever met without a line."

It would be much later that year before Mary found out that, although Robby didn't have a line, so to speak, he had done some covering up of his own. He'd allowed her to assume his upbringing had been like hers. On many occasions Mary mentioned how poor the people in middle Tennessee had been, how "backwards" they were with their horses and buggies and their attitudes. Often, he'd remark with "bless their hearts," allowing Mary to assume that he held compassion for them but certainly nothing in common.

Robby kept up the façade of playing the dapper southern gentleman with fine manners and means. At this point, he wasn't about to tell her that he shared much more affinity with those "downtrodden" Tennesseans than with her, economically anyway. He was sure that she was a fine gal, but to admit his family was poverty-stricken, that just wasn't prudent after having known her less than 10 days.

Apparently, she wasn't finished with her habit of making assumptions, as evidenced with her creating an ideal upbringing for Robby despite having no real evidence to support such a narrative. In fact, based on merely two observations, Mary concluded that Robby's family background was like hers. First, she had overheard him talking with Alabama about blue-blood families that the two southerners both knew. And when Mary had asked Robby what his mother Sara's maiden name was, without boasting, he said it was Marshall, adding that she was a direct descendant of Chief Justice John Marshall's brother and was "some kind of distant cousin to George Marshall."[4] So, without delving further, she decided that he must be well heeled, and soon saw no harm in asking him if he could lend her 100 dollars.

By the time it was announced that they were approaching Liverpool, the prospect of a shopping spree had sprouted in Mary's mind. Somehow, she forgot there was a war on and figured that very soon (since they were now on *this* side of the pond) she would be able to get over to Paris and buy a dress and maybe a bottle of perfume.

With no hesitation, Robby doled out the money and told her that it wouldn't be necessary to pay him back, discreetly chuckling at the notion of Mary frolicking about Europe and spending money like a pre-war tourist.

In her service diary, Mary penned:

> February 19, 1944
> Our last nite on board ship, and I feel like crying because I just parted from the most wonderful fellow in the world. He's made this voyage paradise for me. He says he loves me more than I'll ever know, and the feeling is so mutual. We are hoping that we will be able to be together in England. I just spent the most wonderful 2 hrs. of my life on deck, with the sweetest rebel American soldier there ever was. I'm very sleepy and besides I want to dream so will have to shut this little book for tonite.

The HMS *Andes* docked at the port of Liverpool. It took all day to sort out which troops on board would go where, so Mary and Robby ended up having one more full day together before the 39th's nurses were taken to various private homes in Altrincham, a town in Trafford, Greater Manchester.

In another note from her service diary, she wrote:

---

4   George Marshall, the U.S. Army's Chief of Staff, 1939–1945, won the Nobel Prize for Peace in 1953 and was said to be a descendant of John Marshall, Fourth Chief Justice of the United States, famous for his decision in Marbury vs. Madison.

February 20, 1944

Stayed on board all day and spent every moment from 8 a.m. to 8:30 p.m. with the one I love more than I can say. I didn't cry when I left him because I'm so certain that he will come to me in England. Debarked at 10 p.m. via 6×6 to train in Liverpool, arrived at our destination about 1 a.m. To bed at 5 on straw bunks…

Up at 6:45—finally settled in private homes. The English call it "billeting." Mona and I are together in a lovely British home and have been treated very generously. Have no idea how long our stay is to be but are enjoying our comforts while we have them. Wrote a letter to Robby today and hope he gets it very soon. Walk to meals about 7 blocks away. Spent the evening with the Buckley family in front of the fireplace—discussed the war, the "Battle of Britain," etc. It's very interesting to hear our allies' views of the situation. All I can say is that I'll be so very thankful when it's over and we can return to our loved ones once more. Thank goodness Mona is with me. We can take anything together. The evening ended with cocoa and English cakes which were very good…

CHAPTER 11

The Buckleys

The Buckley home was located on one of the prettiest lanes in Altrincham, just off the town square. Mona had grown up in an Iowa farmhouse, "almost as plain as a barn," she told Mrs. Buckley the day she caught Mona studying the stylistic intricacies of her Tudor home.

Heavy oak paneling rose from the baseboards up the walls reaching over six feet in height, meeting a wide ledge that jutted to separate the panels from the cerulean-painted walls above. The sections of paneling were three feet wide, the centers of each containing unique three-dimensional carvings. Some were of botanical scenes; others displayed symbols from the Far East like a little Buddha or a pond of lotus flowers. Except for the kitchen, all the downstairs living areas boasted the paneling, culminating with the grand fireplace's panel rising above the mantel and displaying the Buckley family crest. There were red Persian rugs with hints of the same blue on the walls above the panels. In the dining room, a hutch held a 15th-century silver tea setting from Mrs. Buckley's side of the family. Mona was in awe.

The balding Mr. Buckley looked a bit like a leprechaun with his diminutive stature and green Sunday suit. But what a jewel he was, insisting that the nurses not touch any of their belongings. He staggered and bumped about the stairs all on his own to haul the army trunks, duffel bags, boxes, and suitcases to the guest quarters. Between huffed breaths, he commented that he wasn't certain that the army was going to allow that much excess to be dragged to war. Even if he didn't understand the American way of life, he certainly appreciated the American GIs and their absolute determination to help his country defeat the Nazis. His wife had talked him into volunteering to house the nurses, and already he was happy to have them.

After having spent most of the past winter wearing those itchy woolen stockings and army khakis, the nurses of the 39th were delighted to hear that standard issue while in England would be the brown and white seersucker dresses. Mrs. Buckley thought them to be "absolutely adorable." Mona and Mary longed for a mother figure even though they had been through a year of rigorous army life. They instantly depended on Mrs. Buckley for advice and support, and although Mary and Mona found most of the English in Altrincham to be a "bit stand-offish" at first, they soon began to see how warm the Brits really were. Mary realized that their sense of decorum may have been misunderstood by Americans. In addition, the Brits had been under attack from the Germans for years. What culture could survive such a beating and not come off a bit aloof and perhaps a little untrusting? Mary wrote to her father that she was "beginning to realize the full meaning of war when I see what these people are going without, how their homes, etc., have been bombed. I hope everyone in the U.S. realizes how fortunate they are to have what they do and not have to worry about being bombed out. These people are carrying on beautifully and one can't help but have the deepest admiration and respect for them. I'd be ashamed to admit how scared I am at night every time I hear a plane or a strange whistle blow."

After a few days of orientation at the 39th's headquarters, the nurses were given two days to organize their belongings in their billeted homes. Mary's original tennis racquet was long gone, but when Mr. Buckley told her about the grass tennis courts nearby and that they were meant to open just as soon as the winter left them for good, she managed to purchase a new one, or at least a slightly used one, the day she and Mona walked to town to look for bicycles. The racquet was just a few pounds, and she still had that money that Robby had given her. Even though Mona didn't play tennis, Mary knew she would find the time and someone to hit a few balls with. And the difference in the sum for renting the racquet as opposed to buying it was so minimal that she decided to buy the racquet outright.

They arrived back at the Tudor house gliding down the lane on their rented bicycles. Mrs. Buckley waved both of her arms and smiled joyfully. She looked pleased to witness the two young women enjoying themselves on their street. As Mary gazed at Mrs. Buckley on the walk in front of her house, something about her image reminded her of the photograph of Robby's mother that he had shown Mary when they were still on the *Andes*. Mary had commented to him that his mother looked as small and tiny as a child and that she looked as thin as a paper doll. So, too, was Mrs. Buckley, and Mary imagined that if Mrs. Buckley were to ever unhinge that tightly constructed bun on the back of her head, a long and silky auburn train of hair would possibly prove to be longer than the length of the middle-aged woman's entire body. Robby had told Mary that his mother's hair also was reddish brown, so she suspected that Mrs. Buckley and her future mother-in-law shared a common Scotch-Irish ancestry.

Mrs. Buckley maintained a tightly composed manner, but when she was exceptionally joyous her blue eyes danced about. She told Mary and Mona that Derek, their only child, would be coming for an extended weekend, and he would be quite happy to romp about town on his bike with the two lovely American ladies. And, to Mary's delight, she said that he would be "ecstatic" to play tennis with Mary.

Mona whispered to Mary that she was dying to take a closer look at the Victorian oil paintings with those gilded frames that hung above the paneling in the living areas. It would take a ladder to get close enough to really study them, but she was far too shy to ask Mr. Buckley if she could borrow a ladder. Mona's first love wasn't nursing. She was an artist, but her practical mid-western background would never have allowed so risky a vocation.

Mrs. Buckley soon grew so fond of Mona that she insisted that after the war she would take her to some of the most beautiful Tudor manors in the English countryside. And then they would go to London and see Buckingham Palace. She would give Mona a pencil sketch book if she promised a return visit when "this country gets right into shape again," adding, "it won't take us long I assure you, now that your American boys are here."

While Mona appreciated the decor, Mary noticed the smell of the house. Each time she entered she would take in a pleasurably long inhalation and say, "Golly, this home always smells so good—like a mix of juniper berries and lilacs." But her favorite part of the house was the casement window in the bedroom that she shared with Mona. Its interior ledge was so deep that she could sit in it with her legs crossed and peer out one of two clear windows that flagged a massive center window made of leaded glass.

Below, the gardens were arranged in squares and rectangles. That spring she often watched the Buckleys' gardener checking the patches of dirt that Mrs. Buckley hoped would soon hold myriads of tulips, but this spring she couldn't guarantee it, as England was enduring an unusual drought. Since 1940, the gardener reserved one raised section for vegetable planting. Virtually every Allied household raised vegetables since supply routes from the Mediterranean had been cut severely ever since Hitler invaded Poland in 1939.

Mary hoped that rain would finally show and entice the tulips to bloom, and that the unit wouldn't be called to the war before she got to see the reds and yellows thrive. While such a beautiful home life made Mary happy, it also saddened her, as the Buckley home became a daily reminder of her real

St. Paul family. She spent the fifth night in England on the casement window's massive ledge weeping and sniffling, folding her body into a ball and rocking forward and back. When would life ever be the same? It wouldn't. Mary squinted her teary eyes and forced them to look out the window and peer at the Altrincham sky. Better she shouldn't think about St. Paul. It was now as far away as the unnamed stars that touched the night sky and then vanished, as if they'd never existed at all.

***

The next morning, she woke to a gentle tapping on her shoulder.

Mona asked her if she'd been in the window all night. Her eyes were swollen. She must have cried herself to sleep there. Never made it to the bed.

Mary was blue, missing St. Paul more than ever.

Mona brought a tea service up to their room. There was nothing to do that day. The Buckleys were busy with tasks out in the country, foraging for eggs and the like. Each family was allowed one fresh egg per week. One dried egg packet was allotted every four weeks. Mrs. Buckley had saved three packets to be consumed in anticipation of the girls' arrival. Today they were hoping to secure a hen from a farm that belonged to some friends. Otherwise, fowl was almost impossible to get. And sugar rations had been so strict that they had resorted to honey only on the tea service. Mary didn't mind that. She preferred honey over sugar in her tea.

Their room was getting chilly. A small fire waned, so Mona moved a corner table in front of the fireplace. She said they'd take their tea there.

The gardener brought up more wood. Soon it caught and crackled. Clouds were forming, but he said not to get overly hopeful. In past years, those clouds already would have produced rain. This spring, they were merely a mirage.

By the second cup of tea, their feet warmed. Mona insisted that Mary talk about her melancholy. She reminded Mary that she was five years her senior and had learned that holding in the blues made them so much worse. Better she should talk it out.

Mary felt conflicted. She loved the security, the comfort, really, that the Buckleys' hospitality and home allowed them. She had found the love of her life in Robby. There was no reason to feel so blue. She was ashamed to even admit to the melancholy.

Mona countered. She found transitions to be the hardest, and certainly their stint in England would count solely as a mark on the calendar, a bridge, between peace and chaos. Maneuvers were rough, yes, but only a war simulation. There were so many questions. When the crossing of the Channel would finally come. Would the 39th be part of the first wave to drive the Germans out of France? Would Mary get to see Robby again before the invasion? So many questions left unanswered and yet the answers would directly impact their lives. Some of those answers might destroy their hopes and dreams. There were no guarantees of anything anymore. Hell, the Buckleys couldn't even guarantee that they would come home with a hen or another fresh egg. They'd been living this life for two years now, waiting for help from the American forces. Their transition had been awfully long, and yet they figured out how to have fun in spite of everything.

"How they joke and carry on," Mona said. "You love it every time Mr. Buckley teases us—the one about American GIs—overfed, oversexed, and over here."

Mary smiled a bit. She did love that joke.

Mona reached across the table to hold Mary's hands. Secretly, she feared that Mary had taken on too much emotionally. She didn't for the life of her understand why Mary would go against the promise to herself that she'd stay away from men and then immediately fall for a tanker on the way to war. It was nonsensical. A tanker, for God's sake. He was wonderful. But they'd been through training on tank injuries. So brutal. There were 2,000 men on that boat, and she chose a tanker. On top of that, she hadn't even broken things off with Zim. There were three letters from him on the desk.

Out loud, Mona asked her if she wanted a third cup of tea.

She didn't. She thought a nap might help. She hadn't slept much in the window seat.

Mary got up from the little table and walked toward her bed. The counterpane and fresh starched linens were so inviting. Didn't Mona think that a nap would help?

She did, but she added that from now on, she was going to make it a point to not allow Mary to brood. Staying active was key. After all, there was much to explore in this beautiful country. And even though there were no patients to take care of during the wait to cross the Channel, soon they would be needed to help organize medical supplies that were arriving every day.

Mary wound herself tightly into the covers. Wait, was that thunder she heard?

Mona moved toward the window.

"Well, I'll be damned. It's raining."

She stood by the window in awe of the rain. The gardener had been so sure that the mottled clouds were just playing tricks on them again. Looking back, though, didn't Mary share the idea that five months in middle Tennessee now seemed like a week, even though while they were undergoing the experience it felt like it would never end? Then the Atlantic crossing felt the opposite, like time had expanded. New York to Liverpool took a mere 10 days, but didn't it seem to Mary as if they'd been on that ship for a year? But now it was over, and Mary didn't know when she might see Robby again. They had so much to plan, and yet, they were at the mercy of waiting. The war hadn't even begun for them. Waiting for the inevitable hell that war would surely bring—was there anything harder than that? It was the most natural thing to feel blue. Mary had every right to feel it.

Mary didn't answer. She hadn't heard anything since the thunder.

Mona crept to the bedroom door, but it creaked and woke Mary for a moment.

She lifted her wooly mound of black hair off the pillow. With eyes closed, she called out softly, "Mona, do wake me if Robby rings, won't you?"

"Sure, Mary. I was just on my way downstairs so that I could hear the phone. Rest. Remember what Alabama always says—'everything's gonna be alriiiiight.'"

But as she closed the door, she knew the odds were against it.

CHAPTER 12

A Doctor Captain

The doctor captain wallowed in a self-assuredness that reminded Mary of Robby. He looked older, though, possibly close to 40. His receding hairline allowed a display of three deep lines running across his forehead, and his blond, thick eyebrows were unusual, since blonds didn't usually have such pronounced eyebrows. His eyes were a stunning Mediterranean blue and his eyelashes so plentiful that, from a distance, it looked as if he had applied mascara.

He joined Col. Bracher, Major Scanlon, Mary, and Mona for lunch. Major Scanlon introduced him.

Captain Henry Wojtowicz preferred to be called "Captain W." It was easier in medical emergencies to call out "Captain W," he said, and he didn't especially enjoy the medical teams' mispronunciations of his surname. Going by one initial kept his ears from hurting.

He stood about 6'3–4", towering above Major Scanlon. He was a large man in stature, muscular, Adonis-like. Major Scanlon loomed large only in their minds.

The nurses worshipped the major and Colonel Bracher for their fair treatment, their respect for the nurses, their protection of them. Colonel Bracher had been determined to keep the nurses busy during the billeting phase. Without patients to care for, he knew their minds stirred with anxiety over their knowledge of what was coming. One of his biggest responsibilities was to uphold morale. And he needed them to help the enlisted personnel. There was much to do to prepare for the crossing. Every medical supply had to be inventoried. Blood transfusion kits had to be counted and packed, blood bottles, antibiotics, myriads of bandages all crated and labeled correctly. Still, they had no idea when the invasion would take place, nor exactly where.

After lunch, Mona and Mary took their place on the assembly line. The packing was mindless. Mona and Mary acknowledged how much they missed nursing.

"Strange," Mona said. "The next time we have patients it will be somewhere in a war zone."

Mary looked around for her least favorite person in the unit. She didn't see hide nor hair of Chiefee. Nothing made her happier. Mona said that she overheard that Chief Maxson was traveling—she was undergoing some kind of training from another unit. She'd be back in a few days.

To change the subject before someone overheard her disparaging remarks about Chief Maxson, Mary offhandedly asked Mona if she thought he looked like a blond Clark Gable.

Mona knew that Mary was referring to Captain W. It was an apt description. She supposed he did, rather. But the question set her off. She chose to pack the remaining boxes without uttering another word to Mary.

She spent one afternoon lost in thought that maybe she'd given Mary the wrong advice. To cure Mary's melancholy, Mona had told her to stay active, to date other officers, even though Robby had asked Mary not to. She should ignore that request from Robby. After all, what men considered might happen on dates and what women made sure didn't happen was vastly different. Mary was trustworthy. Devoted to Robby. She wouldn't cheat on him. But she was a social creature. If she stayed in the Buckley billet all the time, she'd go nuts. Since Robby had only known her 10 days on the *Andes*, he may not have appreciated how loyal she was.

Mary had interrupted and said that it wasn't that Robby didn't trust her. He didn't trust men.

Sure, that made sense to Mona. But she still felt that Mary should be herself and socialize. It was safe to go out with colonels and majors and captains. And they were always with other couples. It wasn't a big deal, really. Robby wouldn't understand, but she would vouch for Mary if he ever had doubts. After all, she was the one who had to suffer while Mary continually whined, "Oh, if I could just see Robby."

That had made Mary chuckle.

"Oh, ha, ha. I know I'm pathetic. But wait until you fall in love, Mona. It's the worst, best, topsy turvy, silly, most tragic thing in the world."

But that conversation was a month ago. Now things had changed. Mona was growing perturbed.

Derek had been to the Buckley home a few times. He was 18, naïve, and love struck—for Mary. As soon as he met her it was obvious.

Mona realized that Mary didn't see it. But because she didn't recognize Derek's crush, she carried on in her usual Mary way and was accidentally flirtatious with him. Mona's intuition was screaming that there would be consequences. The Buckleys were head over heels in love with that only son. Good Lord. If they had an inkling that Derek was fantasizing about Mary, the shit would fly. They'd blame her. Derek could do no wrong.

Now, on top of the potential Derek powder keg, Mona saw the way that Captain W had ogled Mary. Good God, was any man immune? It was absurd.

Even Col. Bracher's comment to Mary at lunch incensed Mona.

"Oh, Mary, you're such a good storyteller. I sure hope you're taking the time to write down all these experiences." Blah, blah, blah.

A tinge of guilt stirred Mona when she looked over at Mary. She was pouting, no doubt because of Mona's silence. How anyone could be so smart as a nurse and so dumb with social interactions—God, it was annoying. She should explain to Mary why she was mad. But something held her back. It wasn't the right time. Other nurses were packing right beside them. She didn't want to embarrass her. Besides, maybe Mary would figure it out on her own, the Derek thing at least. And the doctor captain. It wasn't a given that he'd be around much. If he was as skilled a surgeon as Col. Bracher had boasted, then he'd probably come and go between units once they were over the Channel. One could only hope. He'd already asked where the girls were billeted. Men swarmed around Mary like flies to honey. Jeez.

***

The next two months allowed Mary to see Robby twice. But after both times, her melancholy worsened. Mona grew increasingly concerned but also continued to be annoyed by Mary's friendliness to the opposite sex. It was like she was holding a grenade of trouble in her tiny hands, especially where Derek was concerned.

In early May, Mary and Derek spent a Saturday afternoon playing tennis. Something had gone terribly wrong. Mona never asked for details. They didn't matter. All she knew was that Derek had made an inappropriate move and because Mary never saw it coming, she hadn't been prepared. She blew her top.

In a furious frenzy, they rode their bikes separately back to the Buckley billet, but Derek beat Mary home. Mr. Buckley had to pry it out of him, but by the time Mary arrived, it had been decided that the gals should find a new billet. Derek would be home for the summer. It wasn't going to work for the girls to be there, too. They'd call Chief Maxson in the morning to ask for Mary and Mona to be housed elsewhere.

By Sunday afternoon, a car picked them up. A sentry loaded their belongings, although most of what they'd brought to the Buckleys' had been shipped back to the States already, per orders from Chief Maxson to lighten their loads before the Channel crossing.

Their new billet was small. The Lehr family consisted of a mother and daughter. Mona was certain that Chief Maxson sought a billet where there was no chance that a young man would be swooning.

"Good call on her part, don't you think, Mary?" Mona said, sardonically.

Mary apologized profusely. She wanted to explain what happened with Derek. Mona said she wasn't in the mood to hear it. The pattern was always the same with Mary.

Incredulous, Mary asked, "What do you mean? What pattern?"

She'd never seen Mona so sarcastic. Obviously, she'd been harboring something for months. She recalled the way she'd acted that day they packed supplies. So quiet. And she'd never explained her mood. Had Mona been carrying something around that long? She should just come out with it already. No harm now, after all. The good times with the Buckleys were over. All they had to look forward to was the war, for God's sake.

Mona realized that her main reason for not telling Mary about Derek's crush or Captain W's obvious attraction for her was fear that Mary would misinterpret her concerns. She would accuse Mona of being jealous. And truly, Mona wasn't jealous. She didn't want to be burdened with all those men. Life was complicated enough. Mona didn't borrow trouble. Mary borrowed it, borrowed it again, and continued to borrow it until the debts mounted to an all-out fiasco and everyone around her had to pay for the borrowing. That was the problem. She knew things were going to blow at the Buckleys'. The fact that Mary hadn't a clue was just scary. No wonder Robby had asked her not to date anyone. Maybe he knew her better than she knew herself.

Mary cried foul. Mona had been encouraging her to date. And those dates had nothing to do with the Derek blow-up. So, she failed to see the connection.

"The Derek situation is just a symptom, Mary. The real problem is that you purposely complicate your life. You do it over and over again. I saw you today, packing all those letters from Zim. You still haven't even written him to say that you're planning to marry Robby! Hell, in your room at Wood you kept a picture of Clinton on your nightstand when you had fallen in love with Zim. You can't let anybody go. Do you realize that? You never let anyone go, and the men just pile up. And don't defend yourself about

Clinton. You didn't let him go, either. The only reason he's not writing you letters is because he found that blonde in Boca. Otherwise, you'd just stack his letters in a pile along with Zim's and Robby's and God knows who else's. Probably the doctor captain. It's crazy. You wonder why you're so depressed? You're depressed because you're not honest with these men. Figure out who you're going to be with and let go of everyone else. Then maybe you won't be dragging me into all your shit."

***

The two didn't interact with each other for the next couple of days. They both fell asleep in a huff and woke in the same huff. Soon enough, though, nurses' duties in England precluded any time for pining away over having been ousted from the Buckleys. They went on challenging hikes with 30-pound packs on their backs. On many days they reported to the unit to help with sorting and packing more supplies, heard lectures on shock, neuro psychiatry, and anesthesia, and watched more films on Nazi aircraft and what to expect once the Allied invasion occurred.

A reprieve in training, with an amusement park visit in which they rode the "Bob", offered them a chance to begin healing. The drought finally lifted late that spring, and by the time they had marched several hikes in heavy English rains and shivered together during lectures, they were close to forgetting the incident.

By the time of the Normandy invasion on June 6, 1944, Mona lay aside any persisting resentment toward Mary once and for all. Mary knew she was fully forgiven when Mona said that if there was any nurse she wanted by her side when it was their turn to cross the Channel and face the war, it was Mary.

The 39th received a potent dose of the typhoid vaccine in preparation for living in France. Mary wrote to her parents that her arm was "as sore as a boil" from the hypo and that all the unit was symptomatic with headache, chills, and nausea. On the day prior to the shot, the unit had been ordered to hike 12 miles, and right after the injection, they walked two more miles in a cold, drenching rain to view more training films. The bedraggled bunch arrived at headquarters in wet fatigues to watch the films, their miserable state a harbinger for the next year and a half they would spend on the Continent.

PART III

European Theater of Operations, Summer 1944

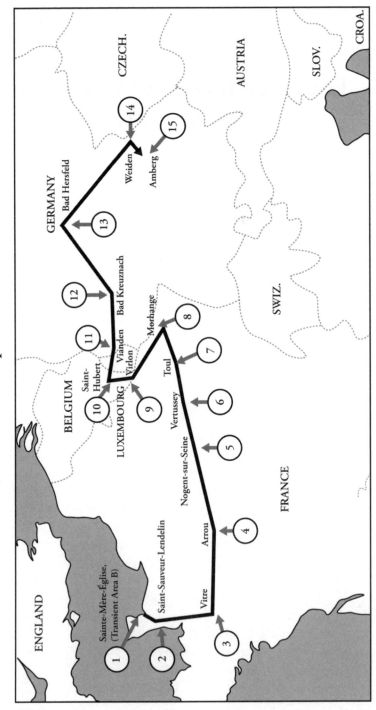

39th Evacuation Hospital's route, 1944–45

Christmas in July

On marshy pillows of green, the dead lay everywhere. It had been six weeks since the Allied invasion of Normandy, but on its roadsides, sycamores, sweet chestnuts, and English oaks clung to the remains of paratroopers who had missed their landing sites. When dawn struck on the first full day of the 39th's arrival, July 19, 1944, Col. Bracher and a few enlisted men combed the area in a jeep, Bracher ordering his driver to stop each time one of them caught sight of a trapped comrade. A PFC volunteered to climb. A ritual commenced—the living boy muttering some prayer to whatever god he worshipped as he cut the dead boy from the confines.

The summer had been so rainy that each body succumbed to the morass with barely an audible thump. As the corpse was released, families of flies that had intermingled with the tangled corpse and chute scattered for a few seconds, their feast interrupted. Soon, though, they re-established their feeding on the ground, the descent carrying one tinny, awful note produced from their collective wings.

In contrast, the evac's preoccupation lay solely with taking care of those still alive. The hanging dead didn't stand a chance to get the attention they deserved. Even the terrain refused to resonate with a thud as a way of offering a unifying despair. Pathos belonged solely to those who watched boys cutting down other boys from soundless trees, stalwart and perfunctory.

The night before, the nurses had crossed the Channel on a liberty ship under blackout conditions, then rode convoy in mostly 6×6 trucks. Eight miles inland, they arrived at Transient Area B, a holding area deemed "safe enough" for evacuation hospitals such as the 39th to gather personnel and supplies and wait for orders. The 39th Evacuation Hospital joined the war

6 June 1944 — D-Day
Our armies landed in Normandy
today and the 2nd front is on.
The day we've been waiting for
and yet dreading as we know
our losses will be heavy.

effort the same day that Operation *Goodwood* began, the Allied battle plan that followed Operation *Overlord*.[1]

Goodwood's mission seemed a "good" one—British and Canadian forces engaged five German divisions in battle on the eastern flank so that the Americans could drive south toward Falaise, employing the 11th and 7th Armored Divisions and the Guards' Armored Divisions. But *Goodwood* didn't go as planned. Germans were able to see the tanks rolling toward them on an eternal expanse of wheat fields as they hid behind camouflaged gun pits. And Allied reconnaissance proved wrong in reports that the Bourguebus Ridge was no longer in German hands, resulting in a deadly pyre of Sherman tanks, 16 of them lost on July 18.

On saffron knolls of wheat, grey walls of destroyed Shermans roasted. Stubborn and orange, the fires serried, flanking black clouds. By Wednesday, July 19, all of Normandy fell under a siege of thunderstorms that seemed almost tropical because of their hurricane-like conditions, dampening the inferno from burning tanks but worsening soldiers' ability to crawl across the scarred terrain seeking dead comrades to be piled on jeeps for later identification. Caen and the Bourguebus Ridge finally were taken from the enemy, but Allied casualties stood at 122,000. And geographically, the Allies had been unable to penetrate Normandy's interior past a 30-mile mark.[2]

Northwest of Caen, the 39th's nurses were ordered to sleep on the ground. It didn't make sense to set up tents with bedding just yet since they had not heard exactly where Colonel Bracher and the first group from their unit had been sent. The skeleton group had left a couple of days before and consisted

1   Rick Atkinson, *The Guns at Last Light*, New York: Henry Holt and Company, 2013, pp. 123–33.
2   Ibid., pp. 134–37.

15 July 1944
Quite late P.m. and we are still waiting on our unit orders. It's getting hard as we can only leave unit blackout for mess and the chow line is at least 3 blocks long. There were several raids during the nite and this A.m. was awakened by one that dropped close as the barracks shook something awful. Ate dinner & July

16th July 1944
Up at 4:30. Left camp at 7. Boarded HM ship at noon 130 nurses quartered in a very small room. Given British complete rations & cot. Marg and I slept on a raft on the deck but spent most of the nite watching the big searchlites follow the planes overhead.

17 July 1944
Still on the channel. Many of the girls are very seasick, but I feel fine. Marg and I invited to dinner by two British officers. First hot meal in 2 days. Debarked at 6 P.m. into small landing boats. Landed on the Utah beachhead at 6:30. Sat in the sand and watched the interesting activity on all sides - the huge number of ships in the harbor with the barrage balloons was a sight I'll never forget. About an hour later boarded trucks and were taken to an area outside St. Germain. Saw many funny pillboxes, the ruins of a church which a few weeks before had held 8 snipers. Slept on the ground after eating our rations for supper. It was cold as we only had 1 blanket but went we were so exhausted slept anyway.

of a few engineers, corpsmen, etc., who were charged with preparing the area by setting up the tents in the form of a cross and performing all the usual tasks they had been trained to do in Tennessee each time the 39th moved during maneuvers training.

Despite their present circumstances, many recalled the time of lavish sleeping in fine English billets and used those memories to entice rest. And they'd come to understand that there was a certain irony that accompanied abnormal circumstances. Whenever the army imposed upon them some uncomfortable living condition, other larger forces would naturally come into play, allowing the original nuisance to shrink instantly by comparison. This time, no tents and minimal bedding seemed hardly problematic when one considered the other environmental forces at work: crackers had been their only sustenance for the last 15 meals; their sopping wet feet had not felt a change of socks or shoes for four days; the war sounds were so pervasive that it was difficult to even hear the orders Chief Maxson barked. Engine sounds of Luftwaffe planes purred distantly and then roared with Doppler sounds of "eeeeyowww" as they flew directly over the vulnerable position of the 39th. The nurses had been so thoroughly trained in the identification of enemy aircraft that they all knew the difference between a Focke-Wulf Fw-190 and a Messerschmitt

Bf 109. They also knew that the Focke-Wulf was often referred to as "The Shrike," nicknamed after the bird that hunts by finding vulnerable prey in a field, dives down to take the poor creature in its beak, and then thrashes the thing against the barbs of wired fences.

PFCs had been part of the first group to cross the Channel a few days ahead of the medical staff and had dug an adequate supply of foxholes at Transient Area B for the remainder of the 39th to camp. Mary, Mona, and Alabama spotted a compromised fox hole to share, the persistent rains having caved in the hole's depth to half its original size. Fortunately, Alabama had grabbed a second blanket, so they used that one to serve as a barrier between them and their bed's foundation, a sheen of cold and pliable mud that caked under the weight of them as they bore down. Mona and Alabama claimed their spots in the mud hole while Mary searched frantically for her helmet. By the time she found it and joined them, she was glad that she was third in the hole as their body heat had warmed the space.

Ordered to remain in the holes with their helmets on, they attempted hopeless positions for sleep. Alabama wryly commented that there wasn't any way that Mary could follow the "helmet-on-head order" since she was still in possession of the one with the burned-up straps. Mary harped back that she guessed the army had a little more going on lately than worrying about replacing her helmet. She added that she really didn't care if the helmet did fall off because all she could concentrate on was her teeth chattering, her body shaking, and her mind reeling about where Robby might be.

Mona took advantage of a couple of seconds between blasts to whisper to Mary and Alabama. She suggested that before they tried to go to sleep, they should help each other peel off their wet shoes and socks. An elated Mary agreed and immediately began to feel about for Mona's shoelaces, her fingers crawling toward the top of Mona's right boot. After she pried off the first boot, she propped Mona's naked foot on to a Val-Pack to prevent it from dropping on to a muddy place in the hole that had not been covered sufficiently with the extra blanket.[3] After both feet were propped on the Val-Pack she liberally smothered them with foot powder. Then she handed Mona a fresh dry pair of socks and her overshoes. The mud-caked boots could be cleaned the next morning. Mona followed Mary's lead, returning the favor by pulling at Mary's wet shoelaces and repeating the process. They nervously giggled at the thought of such an uncanny irony—how they could focus on tugging at each

---

3   A Val-Pack was a small olive drab piece of luggage meant for carrying army uniforms and supplies.

other's muddy boots when the ground beneath them shook and bellowed. Glint of light, then darkness, then boom, then repeat. Light, dark, boom. And in between—rapid clashes—pop, pop, pop, tat-a-tat, tat. Then a flash of light again, less than a second long, then darkness, then the refrain of the cymbal sounds, supported by the continual bass vibrations of the land mines' growling rumble. Soon they'd accomplished an efficient ritual of the drying of feet, despite the mud beneath them and the interminable undersong above, below, and beside.

When they settled themselves sufficiently, Mona slid the flashlight to the off position to follow blackout conditions. By some small miracle, they were asleep by the time Chief Maxson performed bed check.

On the morning of July 19, Chief Maxson announced to the medical personnel that orders were to join their unit at Bricquebec in northwestern France. But no sooner had the men erected the hospital and tents than they received orders to head immediately to Sainte-Mère-Église to relieve the 96th, that evac having been on the Continent for six weeks since the invasion had begun on June 6.

It was when the 39th's medical convoy approached Sainte-Mère-Église that they witnessed the PFCs' grim task of releasing the dead paratroopers. At a distance they also saw what looked like large objects hanging from the trees, but they couldn't make out what in the world the things were. As they got closer, they realized the massive shapes were those of dead cows and horses, macabre ornaments that looked like they'd been hung by Satan, his version of Christmas in July.

The 96th had been responsible for treating the casualties resulting from the Allies taking Sainte-Mère-Église, which had the distinction of being the first French town to be liberated from four years of German occupation. If appearances of the 96th's members were any indication, the 39th's nurses felt an aggregated panic over the realization that *they* were most likely going to look exactly like the 96th looked after *their* first six weeks of war. In a word, the 96th looked like shit.

A lot of the 96th's original patient load had either perished or had been sent back to the fighting. A fraction had been shipped back across the Channel for further surgeries. Most of the 39th's encounters with the 96th weren't during formal briefings but instead were during chow, just for a few meals, before the bedraggled lot convoyed west for some R&R. It was not uncommon to hear nurses from the 96th say they'd lost 20 pounds in those first six weeks. Others talked of the types of wounds they'd treated. Two tent mates recounted a particular morning when they'd been able to grab shuteye for a couple of hours and then had meandered still half-asleep toward Medical Ward. One of them almost tripped on a boot that still housed a soldier's foot and calf. They were certain that they would have noticed it had it been there the night before. Later a corpsman explained. It had belonged to the enemy and, most likely, a Messerschmitt had been blown out of the sky, the applied forces along with an ensuing fire helping to sever its inhabitants' bodies into parts that then plunged to the ground—like "manna from heaven," he said.

CHAPTER 14

Bed-Check Charlie

Somewhere in France
July 19, 1944
Dearest Family,

And I thought maneuvers were rough, but then we weren't prepared for that and we are for this, although it's rather different than I anticipated. Wish I could tell you all about it but everything is snafu as you realize.[1] It's just like 4th of July around here and we just pretend that it is. And at nite when it's rather weird and we're sure it's a Jerry plane we tell each other it's a truck at the same time grabbing our helmets. Last nite we were so tired, the three of us spread a blanket on the ground and one over us and slept the best we have for a week. Survived the trip OK and I didn't have to use the paper sack they gave us before we left. And I feel wonderful except for the 20 layers of dirt accumulated the last week. Just took my shoes off for the first time in 4 days and nites and boy does it feel good. Smothered my feet in foot powder. I drink so much water don't ever have enough to wash with. Soon after we landed were riding in a truck which landed in a ditch, but no one was hurt, and we just laughed. Well, it's beginning to rain so guess I'll put my raincoat on and look for a tree.

Please don't worry. Although there's never a dull moment now, it's not more than we can take. We are more than re-paid for discomforts by the happy looks on the boys' faces when they see us.

Lovingly,
Mary

France
July 21, 1944
Dearest Family,

It's after 11 P.M. and just got my patients settled and will try to write a few lines before more will come. This is the first opportunity I've had to write for a couple days now—so much has happened that my head is whirling. Got caught up on some much-needed rest this P.M. so feel ready feel for anything tonite. We work 7-7 shifts, and I drew "nites," but I don't mind. It's been raining steadily, and we are wearing our arctic boots to keep dry. This life is very familiar to some of us, except that last year it seemed darned futile and this time it's gratifying but frightening too. However, one gets so tired you just sleep thru anything.

---

1   SNAFU was army slang for Situation Normal: All Fucked Up.

It's 4th of July day and nite. Haven't had mail call for a couple of weeks now but sure hope we get some soon... Thank goodness we're so busy and tired we don't have much time to think. Please write often and please keep sending me Kleenex and something to eat.

More later,

Lovingly,

Mary

Somewhere in France

July 23, 1944

Dearest Daddy,

I'm going to try to write a decent letter instead of a note this time. Just haven't had time until now and have been so tired just couldn't write a decent letter. It's Sunday morning and I just got off duty and finished breakfast. We had fresh rolls. They tasted super. Am trying to stay awake until 9:30 for church and then will try to get some shuteye until time for duty again.

Gee, Daddy, if I come home with white hair and look about forty years old don't be shocked because many more nights like last night will make nervous wrecks out of us. It was fairly quiet until about 1 a.m. and then somebody opened a terrific barrage that just about shook the patients out of bed and me—well, I just grabbed my helmet and hit the dirt. Then one of the boys from the other ward came to see if I was scared and he was so scared himself his teeth were chattering. Instead of comforting the patients it was the reverse. They've been right up there, are used to it, I guess. Well, we probably will get used to it, too, and I feel like a coward but will try to overcome my fear so I can at least take a temperature without trembling. And then all the things we see and hear make us want to cry. We feel so desperately sorry for these boys—especially the younger ones, but they're wonderful soldiers, Daddy, and the best patients in the world. I swear I'll never complain about the fact that it's rough living the way we do after talking with boys who've spent days in muddy foxholes. But no matter what they've gone through here, these Yanks just never lose their spirit. Of course, they're pretty shaken up and terribly nervous, but they can still joke and appreciate the swing music we have going from dawn 'til blackout.

This morning everyone came to when they played "Paper Doll" for reveille. Gee, music and mail are about the best morale builders there are for us now. We can't get out of the area and furthermore don't want to so when we can't get recreation Uncle Sam brings it to us and that's the way it will be until our job is finished here. We have a large recreation tent where we have movies, a couple of wonderful radios, phonographs and plenty of pocket-size books for reading material. And of course, a 12-hour work shift doesn't leave much time to brood. Our work is our life now and here's one gal that doesn't care if she has to wear fatigues and leggings for the duration if only this thing gets over and we can get back to the States...

Had mail call yesterday... for most of our patients, it was the first time they've had mail since D-Day.

Finally, the mail brought a stack of letters from Robby.

... Robby's letters just renew all my hopes and faith for the future and are a wonderful inspiration. He says we're getting married just as soon as we hit the home shore and that will make up for all that we are enduring now. Even if we had to be separated for the rest of this old war it's worth being in love with a man like him and having him love me the way he does. I know you and Mom will love him, too, and will think I made a wise choice.

The weather is cold and rainy, and I just wait for the time to come when I can crawl into that wonderful sleeping bag. In spite of the continuous noise don't have much trouble sleeping until they decide to explode some mines and the ground starts to shake like yesterday...

At Sainte-Mère-Église, the majority of the 100 patients inherited from the 96th Evac were German, so those in the 39th with fluency became sought-after and highly regarded. Mary's German proficiencies elevated her status in the unit beyond her reputation as "prettiest pinup gal of the 39th." There were a few unit members who could pick up enough of the German patients' words to interpret how to care for them, but only a handful like Mary could read and write in the language, an invaluable asset for taking care of the German patients, especially those whose war injuries precluded their ability to speak. They could write on an old piece of board or, if the nurse happened to find a piece of paper, a rare commodity, the German boy wrote the message on it. Then a corpsman often searched for Mary to decipher it. And during rare breaks from duty, corpsmen who had previously interacted with Mary by flirtatiously remarking how they "wished" they were officers so that they could ask her "for a date," etc., were, in general, now respectfully asking her to remediate their German slang deficiencies. They admitted, though, that the foreign language phrase they enjoyed saying the most wasn't German at all but rather French. They'd picked it up from the French villagers who continually harangued—"*Allez nous tuer un Allemand*," or, "Go kill us a German."

After having witnessed only two weeks of the sheer mindlessness of war, it's certain that, even though most of their patients were German prisoners of war, the nurses and docs found themselves also muttering the phrase. And, after having heard how the first of their own died on the Continent, the "Go Kill Us a German" slogan evolved from a guilt-ridden echo to a guilt-free mantra.

Somewhere Overseas
July 28, 1944
Dearest Family,
    Am sitting on the ground outside our wigwam. It's a pleasant warm day, but the general atmosphere is morbid. Something awful occurred that has sort of shaken everybody. One of our nurses died last night. Three of them were out with some officers and they got hold of some wine that the Germans had evidently poisoned, although the girl was the only one who suffered the effects. They think she may have aspirated when she was vomiting. Anyway, when they got her to the nearest hospital it was too late. Three of us went for a walk last evening and 3 medical officers drove by us in a jeep and asked us to join them in town. We had some wine too but here's one gal that's never going to touch another drop of the stuff. Didn't get sick cause none of us had very much. We had some salmon sandwiches to go with it—the fellows rations. At least we know better than to eat any food but our own here.
    Chiefee had bed check before we got back, but the kids covered for us. Then after I had gotten to bed the fireworks started again and everyone was up all night and couldn't figure out

why the scaredest one of the bunch slept. That's me. I did wake up once and put my helmet on and sat on the edge of the bed but was so sleepy just dropped off into dreamland again.

Those doctors we were with last night teased the daylights out of me and, as usual, treated me like a child—and thot I was too young to be in the thick of this mess but when I see our young boys feel like a mother to them. Yesterday specialed a severe case of pneumonia. He was just twenty years old and just a beautiful boy and the best patient I've ever had. As sick as he is he always says thank you for every little thing.

Received your letter of the 15th Daddy, the first I've had from the States in three weeks. Sure was glad to hear from you and now am looking forward to those packages that you mentioned Mother is sending. Robby is so darned faithful, and I'm sure I don't know what I'd do without his wonderful reassuring letters. They're heartbreaking, as he's just as lonesome as me. He was so pleased with your letter, Mom, and said it put his mind at ease so much as he said it was so hard to make a good first impression through a letter. In yesterday's letter he said for me to try to remain the same sweet, adorable Mary as when we were together last. Also, that his thoughts and prayers are with me all the hours of the day, etc. I'm so afraid I can't remain the same, though. Seems like this war makes you grow old overnite, but one of our officers said to me yesterday—Mary, you won't grow old if you just keep that beautiful smile and it's very hard to smile sometimes, especially when I get so scared. Gee, our boys call me their girl with the million-dollar smile. I bet you think I'm awfully conceited, but it's those little things that make a girl still believe that life is sweet when there's so much misery all around. You see this morale-building works both ways. I'm sure I don't know what we'd do without our boys in our unit helping us through some of these days. I know half of them are as frightened as we are and yet they're always reassuring us. It's nice to have been with them on maneuvers. We recall those days in Tenn. often and always find something to laugh about. And they're right up to date on my love affairs but don't see why it's always an officer. Of course, I've really only been in love once and still am and always will be now...

Back in February, just before the unit had made the crossing over the Atlantic, Dagny Solberg had whisked about New York City with Mary and Mona. Almost six months later, she served as the charge nurse for the day shift in the Medical Ward tent in Sainte-Mère-Église, briefing Mary that the 20-year-old pneumonia patient was hanging on and that Mary had, once again, been assigned to "special" him closely for the next 12 hours. She added that maybe the Private Redmond would be strong enough for Mary to grab a few minutes to offer him a "spit bath," and a shave. Then Dagny asked Mary about dinner. It was "per Army usual" (dehydrated scrambled eggs) but, on a cheerier note, Mary had heard promises from "chef" that on Sunday there would be "real pineapple pie." She wished Dagny a decent night's rest despite the indecent weather. Thunderstorms continued to commandeer the skies and tonight would likely be accompanied by the usual pops and spatters of artillery fire, explosions, and bomb blasts.

In Normandy, the medical tents were set up virtually the same way they'd been set up during maneuvers, and while the army had designed certain sensible protocols for set-up, really the individual evacs could organize them to their liking. A total of 30 cots, 15 on each side of the tent's walls, allowed enough space for a middle aisle so that medical personnel had room to move a supply cart around as needed. Typically, they would reserve the first two cots closest to the "ward area" for the most critically ill patients. This way they could monitor them closely or grab supplies to re-fill the cart.

In a traditional hospital setting, the ward, of course, is the area in which nurses sit at desks to accomplish their paperwork, confer with each other regarding certain patients over a cup of coffee, greet visitors, and, during Mary's tenure, "bow down" to doctors when they appeared on the scene. The ward area in the tent was similarly designed, but they were lucky if just one stool was available to get off their legs for a minute or two. Usually there was some sort of table serving as a nurse's desk on top of which would be kept a drug formulary and Army Nurse Corps policies and procedure manuals. There was usually an army-supplied jar of peanuts, and Mary was intent to supply the desk with homemade snacks, too, like mocha cakes from "Gram," or popcorn and cookies that Inga sent. Though her mother only used the unsalted popcorn as a buffer to safeguard the cookies from crumbling during transport "over the pond," Mary soon discovered that the staff and convalescing patients enjoyed the stale popcorn almost as much as the cookies even though Inga hadn't intended the popcorn for eating.

The engineers would set up a double-eyed hotplate in the ward area, too, mostly intended for heating water for the patients and brewing coffee for the medical staff, even hot chocolate if they could get it. Medical supplies were held in crates and stacked about in the ward area. In July, there were still many supplies available—boxes of bandages, IV tubing, plasma bottles, water bottles with a couple of small boxes filled with lemon crystals used to add vitamin C. Other crates held medications, and there was usually a small box of candles, some half-melted but still usable and always chosen for a light source over flashlights since blackout conditions were paramount.

Cots were placed only two or three feet apart from each other and were pathetically uncomfortable, but for men who'd lived on the ground they must have seemed plush. Olive drab blankets covered the patients, although the nurses were never satisfied with the number allotted, as patients who suffered from rigors couldn't get warm from one thin blanket. Pillows remained in short supply, too.

Even during the day, the tents were dim, but night duty challenged the medical personnel to know exactly what supplies were kept where since much of their work depended on navigating in an unsympathetically dark environment. Everyone who'd been in maneuvers training had long been accustomed to the conditions, although the tense atmosphere caused by the war sounds reminded the staff that they were no longer hearing friendly fire.

Facing the patients' cots from the ward area, Mary's patient was supine in the first cot on the right. At the foot of the cots, the patients' charts hung. She scanned the chart for his latest vitals that Dag had recorded at 1700.

Under the thin blanket the shape of his bony, taut legs looked like her cross-country skis she'd left in the downstairs closet of "1262." He was napping, but when she approached him to take his temperature, he winced a bit. She muttered how sorry she was that she had to bother him. Her voice had a distinctive quality. Even when she whispered, her pristine elocution held fast, so the private recognized who was hovering above him without opening his eyes. There was a tenderness in their exchange, whispers like "Gee, I'm glad to see my favorite nurse," followed by "Gosh, I'm sorry I have to put this darn cold stethoscope on your chest."

Rattling sounds persisted in haunting his deep breaths, but they weren't as pronounced as the night before last. Still, despite hopeful signs like lighter rattles, sometimes pneumonia made a dirty deal with death behind the caregiver's back. It was still too soon to tell with Private Redmond. At least his youth was in his favor.

Mary handed him a cup of water and dropped in lemon crystals, despite his pleading not to be asked to drink the "nasty-tasting French excuse for H2O."

There was a fine line between giving a pneumonia patient too much water as opposed to not enough when it was obvious that he needed hydration. Too much could cause more fluid build-up in the already compromised lungs.

He didn't have to drink much at all. She'd put in extra lemon crystals. She'd make a deal with him. He would take in two or three sips in the time it was going to take her to heat up water for his bath and shave.

Redmond wanted to know if she'd been able to rest while she'd been off duty, especially with all the visits from "Bed Check Charlie," army idiom for enemy strafing and blasts. A land boom interrupted any answer and shook the ground beneath the Med Ward tent. There were varied forms of "Je—su—s" audible throughout the tent. With blasts of that magnitude, instinct dictated hitting the dirt.

At first, Mary and another night-duty nurse simply crouched, but when the blasts didn't stop, Mary chose to lie flat alongside the private's cot, then reached for the private's hand. The gesture was meant to temper his fear, but his large hand with spindly fingers offered her the calm reassurance that she was trying to offer *him*. Despite his frailty, this response might be another indication that just maybe he was mustering enough strength to beat the pneumonia.

She lay on the ground waiting for any sign at all that the bombs had stopped detonating, or that the planes had left the air space right above them, taking their whirling hums with them. Was it at least five minutes that she lay there, pulsing her hand inside his, squeezing after each sound burst? Finally, there were lighter sounds—intermittent crackles.

During the sequence of heavy blasts, her right ear responded with a feeling of tightness, as if she needed to relieve pressure off the eardrum. Once the sounds became less frequent, she noticed the ringing. For then on, she was never free from that vexing ringing in the right ear.

When the bombardment subsided, she released her hand from the private's soft grip and made her way to the hot plate to heat water. The charge nurse had returned to the ward area, too, and Mary told her that after she got her "special" settled, she'd be happy to help her look after the other patients. As she put the pot of water on the hot plate, she wondered if Captain W might arrive. Even though he was a surgeon, she'd heard that he was covering patients on Medical, too. He may have been trying to catch some shuteye before making rounds. She hoped he'd show. She wanted his opinion about Redmond's condition, hoping that her interpretation of his lung sounds was accurate and that just maybe he'd turned the corner.

She grabbed a candle from a box and returned to Redmond's cot. She dug into her pocket to feel for a matchbook, choosing it over her father's cigarette lighter to light the candle. She couldn't bring herself to burn up the fuel in the lighter. It had become a symbol for home. If possible, she'd always find another source of light. Her other front pocket held her nursing scissors and a bibelot of a tank, the one Robby had given her on the *Andes*. She held it between her forefinger and thumb. Just like the cigarette lighter, the tank served as a talisman. She showed it to the private, telling him that her fiancé was a tanker just like him. After she teased him that it didn't look like he'd done a very good job of drinking the "nasty French water," he moved his dry lips, eked out half a grin. She would remember to chart that the patient's spirits seemed improved.

The charge nurse had positioned the supply cart halfway down the aisle, so Mary took the lit candle to search for washcloths and bar soap, toothbrush and paste, razor, and Glider shaving cream, a popular brand in the early forties. The candlelight died by the time she made it to the cart. She cursed the candle, grabbed the items in the dark, and returned to her patient.

He muttered a bit during the warm "spit bath," but Mary interpreted his faint murmurs as positive responses. The poor boy must have been pleased to feel a hot washcloth touch his face, his underarms, his feet.

She wondered if he had strength enough to wash his private areas on his own.

He said that he'd like to try, so she handed him a clean, warm cloth and secured him as he moved sideways to clean himself.

It was time for a shave. Many of the wounded and sick admitted to the evacs often had long hair and beards, and most carried lice, too. Upon Redmond's admission, he'd been too sick for a trip to the de-lousing station, although Mary hadn't detected any white flakes in what looked to be a full and matted head of auburn, but who knew given the fact that the few times she'd been his nurse the only light available for observation was lackluster at best.

There were promises to have a corporal shave his head and give it a "good scrub" when he felt better, which, from the looks of him, would be "very soon." She lied. The rattles sounded worse again. Had the pneumonia made its deal with death after all? She'd seen it many times. A doc or nurse would be convinced that the patient had turned the corner and then, in an hour's time, the patient would have expired. One never knew.

Would he be up for a good tooth-brushing, she asked.

He needed to sleep, but his heroic nature forced him to shift his body up from the cot just long enough for her to brush his teeth. She dipped the toothbrush in the bowl of warm water. The anemic candle flickered, then extinguished itself for the fourth time. She apologized for the darn candle being so stubborn, and then struggled to re-light it with anxious, harried hands.

He gagged. When she got it lit for the fifth time, there were bubbles, froth, spume of white falling out of his mouth. He looked almost rabid.

The next few seconds were marked with confusion. She grabbed another washcloth to dab the fizz from his cheeks and neck, then handed him a cup to spit. She felt weaker than bath water right after she realized what she'd done.

> … After I finished giving my pt. his bath decided to brush his teeth for him as he was quite weak and darned if I didn't use his shaving cream instead of toothpaste, and he just foamed at the mouth it was so soapy. In the first place I was so sleepy after not getting any rest the evening before and besides it was so dark in the tent couldn't see that it was Glider shaving cream instead of toothpaste…

For the last several mornings at reveille, the 39th's loudspeaker had played "Paper Doll" by the Mills Brothers. After that night shift, Mary began a process of becoming a paper doll herself, discarded and disintegrating in the Norman rains.

CHAPTER 15

Poppies

The subject of the "poppy" field had arisen in a brief conversation with W the night before when he'd brought her a cup of coffee at Private Redmond's bedside. She'd noticed the blooms on the ride to Sainte-Mère-Église, but that was almost two weeks ago, so already she may have missed seeing them at their peak. They weren't poppies, though. This was a misidentification, as in Normandy's seasons poppies would have been over by mid-June. More than likely, by late July, the field Mary had seen was of hawksbeard, asphodel, marjoram, and various and sundry thistle.

The next afternoon, on the 30th, there was a lull in patient load. And the rains that had dictated most of July's weather patterns finally moved out, creating an opportunity for finding that flower field. A pebbled road led Mary and W atop a hill located less than a quarter of a mile from the 39th's position. Below was spread a majestic array of colors both alarming and wondrous. The slight winds caused the flowers to move like graceful, swaying sylphs. That these blooms—delicate, fragile, vulnerable, brief—existed amid the horror that summer had brought struck the two as nothing short of miraculous. The field stood as a bountiful, symbolic paradox, having survived the mid-range bombing attacks, the strafing. And most likely, the Germans had planted mines just beneath the thick stalks and winding roots.

In a matter of seconds, a bewildering awareness of gratefulness, pleasure, purpose, and awe darted about her mind. There was something about the sight of this place that felt surreal, timeless. The splendor—the silence. God knew there'd been so little of that. And this was the first day since they'd been on the Continent that the natural sounds of summer could be heard—small insects and bumblebees. At last, a celebratory absence of barrage echoes. Maybe she'd died. Probably not, because surely heaven doesn't admit guilt, and there was that nagging tug of it for sharing this afternoon with W instead of Robby.

In the recent past she'd recognized that a task at hand could dissipate the guilt, so she pointed the camera toward a poignant display of color, fiddled with the lens, then shot photos with a capricious flare, all of which helped her replace the guilt with a salve of justification.

Maybe she needed the afternoon with W—psychologically speaking. After all, they'd been through so much hell already. So, there was that. And there was this—this minute right now—this reality that felt like it was not reality, not part of the reality that they'd left down the road anyway, the place where the sick, wounded, dying boys were. There was W, so unspeakably gallant. He'd even thought to bring a picnic. She watched him kneel at the meadow's edge, avoiding any misstep onto a potential minefield, extending his long arms and dexterous, competent fingers picking flowers to build a bouquet.

A heaviness calmed her. This rare tranquility of her spirit prompted W to comment that he wished that he could have caught the moment with the camera, without her being aware of him taking her picture, of course. Photos of her typically revealed tight jaws, a hidden top lip, squinting eyes so taut that she looked as if she were *trying* to etch crow's feet onto her face. She acknowledged that she was a bit "high-strung" and that it did feel good to just "be" for a little while. She perched on an old tire that probably once rolled under a tank. As she waited for W to finish the flower-picking, her thoughts recalled the fall of her 15th birthday.

Even though the doctors had told her family that the TB was no longer a threat to her life by age 14, it would be another year before she finally felt healthy enough to walk "outdoors." As a way of commemorating her private celebration of being able to enjoy nature again, she remembered how she'd collected leaves and when she got back to 1262, how she'd pressed the oranges and reds, purples and dark greens into books nestled in her father's library. Probably that was the first year she'd begun the leaf-pressing ritual.

And now in Normandy, the bounding about of nature's insistent virility, the sharp colors and swaying shapes, the incarnate artistry of God that had materialized in the field of "poppies" altogether summoned in her an awareness. She compelled her mind to store the visuals into her memory as if they were leaves that she was pressing between pages in a heavy book. They would become a perfect image that she could see when her eyes were closed, an array of mental furnishings, pleasing and decorative. She would be able to call on them any time the world became too fierce.

But soon, hints of dusk prompted the wrapping of the crumbs and crusts of leftover bread. W's remark that they should get back to post was almost instantly followed by an approaching ambulance. Mary recognized the emergency medic (EM) driving it. He'd been one of the enlisted men who'd asked her a couple of German language questions, even though the medics were given reference cards highlighting common German phrases. After her wave, he stopped and rolled down the window.

The ambulance was hauling three prisoners of war in the back that the EMs had picked up on the roadside. The one that was "wounded real bad," according to one of the medics, was alone on his side of the ambulance. The EM hopped out of the cab and rushed to the back to slide out the gurney that held the unconscious patient for W to assess.

Like most ambulances in war-time Europe, a piece of plywood ran down the middle of the cabin to accommodate more patients. If need be, two or three men could be stacked on one side, two or three on the other. The patients' gurneys were separated by racks (much like stacked racks inside an oven) so that the medic could slide the patients in and out. Of course, many times there were far more wounded than there were ambulances to carry them, so medics and engineers were forever make-shifting just about anything with wheels to transport the wounded. The most ingenious forms of patient mobilization devices had to have been jeeps. At times, they could be seen carrying up to four men on the hood, six inside the cab, even two more men on the tail-end, secured by rope. If they didn't have any rope left, a medic might be seen bent over the back of the jeep holding onto the patients until they reached either a field hospital or an evac unit.

W and Mary took on a quick stride to join the EM at the back of the ambulance. Mary approached the patient's side and felt for a pulse while W checked his wounds. There was significant blood loss. The boy had held his intestines together with his own pistol belt. His face and extremities paled. Death loomed.

Because of W's size, he couldn't easily fit inside the ambulance to monitor the critical patient for the remainder of the ride back to the evac. He suggested that Mary crawl in the ambulance next to the patient, keep his heart rate going with manual compressions ("perfuse him, if necessary," he'd said.) She tossed the "poppy" bouquet and her camera in the front seat between the sergeant and W. Then she crawled into the cramped rear of the ambulance.

It carried a toxic smell, a mix of ammonia from the urine and metal from the blood. The medic huddled back into the other side to guard the two conscious prisoners of war at gunpoint. The ride wouldn't take more than six or seven minutes, but on the way back to post, a menacing reality replaced the equanimity she'd shared with W just before the ambulance had pulled over to fetch them. It didn't seem to her as if there would ever be any "getting away" again.

She thought back to earlier that afternoon—before the hike to the poppies. He'd brought her stationery. She was thrilled. He asked if she wanted to finally see the field of flowers. They'd made it halfway there when she cursed herself for not having brought along her camera, and he'd been so kind to suggest that they hurry back to the tent to grab it. So, they'd raced each other back, and, despite his being almost 20 years her senior, it didn't turn out to be a fair race at all, his long legs loping along with seemingly no effort. Naturally, he beat her back to the tent, then turned around to watch her scampering to catch up.

"Come on, slow poke," he'd teased, and then he'd laughed after she stuck out her tongue at him. By the time they pursued their second walk to the field, she remembered that they had been almost giddy. Then when they topped that hill how they'd marveled at the mystifying colors below.

But just as the sun began dropping away so fast behind the next hill over, the ambulance had appeared and now, here she sat over a dying German boy.

A realization overcame her. Not even a capricious jaunt to shoot pictures of a meadow's flora was allowed to happen as a singular, happy event.

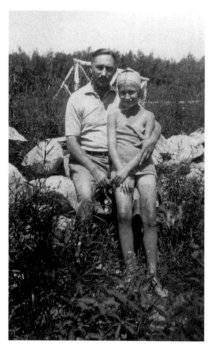

H. C. Balster with his eldest, Bette

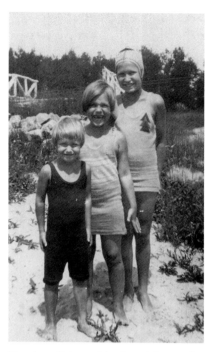

The three Balster girls, from left to right,
Constance, Nancy, and Bette

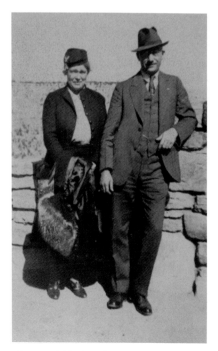

Inga and H. C. Balster in the late 1930s

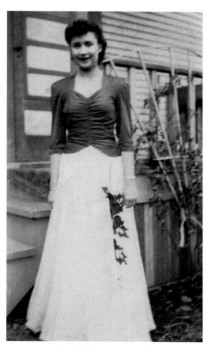

Bette's "sweet sixteen"

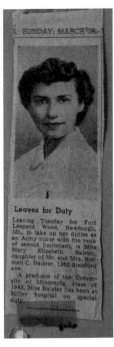

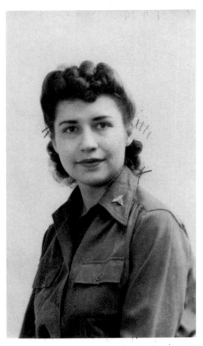

Newspaper announcement of Mary leaving for duty

Second Lieutenant Mary Elizabeth Balster, Ft. Leonard Wood, Missouri

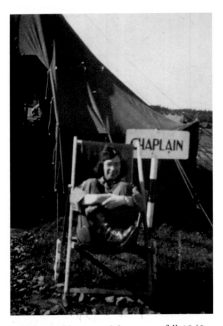

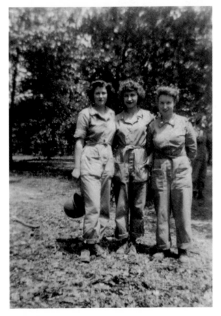

Alabama, Tennessee Maneuvers, fall 1943

From left to right, Lorraine, Mary, and Mona, Tennessee maneuvers, summer 1943

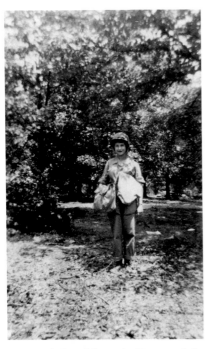

Mary ready for a hike in the Tennessee hills, maneuvers, 1943

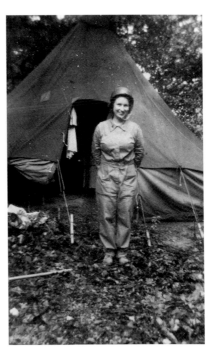

Mona in front of the living quarters tent, Tennessee maneuvers, 1943

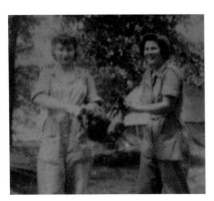

Mary and Lorraine washing fatigues on maneuvers, 1943

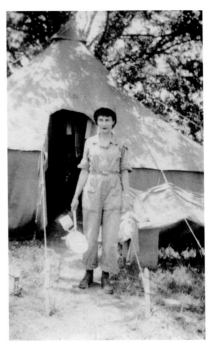

Mary performing daily duties during maneuvers, 1943

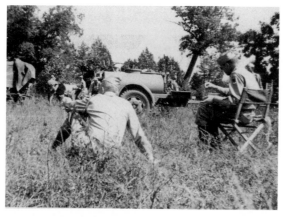

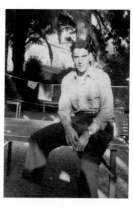

In chair, Colonel Allen Bracher, 1943

Believed to be Lieutenant Hal Zimmerman, 1944

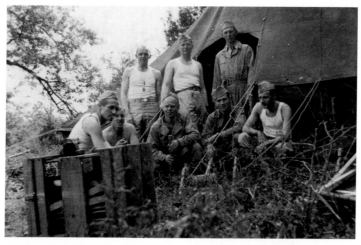

Mary's snap of some of the beloved members of the 39th, from left to right, Capt. Kennedy, MC, Capt. Downing, MC, PFC Bischoff, PFC Ford, E5 Yates, Capt. Michelson, MC, Lt. North, MC, Sgt. Johnson

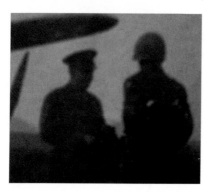

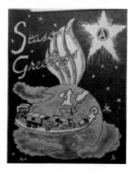

Mary quickly snapped this photo of General Eisenhower talking with General Patton, fall 1944 or spring 1945

Army Greetings card issued by TUSA and sent to every member of Third Army, Christmas 1944

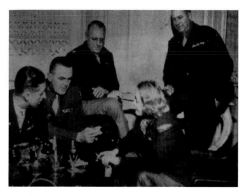

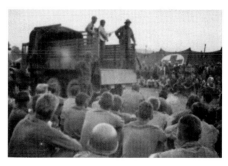

Bing Crosby, center, entertaining the 39th, August 1944

Marlene Dietrich visiting with TUSA Officers, November 1945

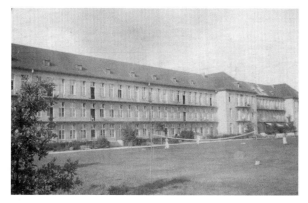

Hospital in Amberg, Germany where Mary worked in the summer of 1945

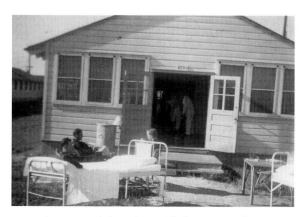

An amputee is brought outside for some sunshine

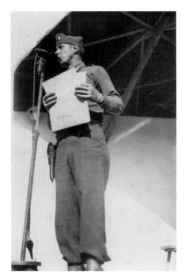

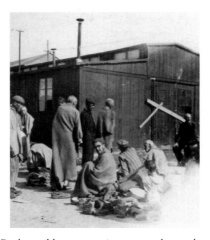

Buchenwald concentration camp, photo taken by Robby. He kept this photo in his wallet until his death at age 88, stating that he "never wanted to forget why we went to war"

Robby giving logistics orders

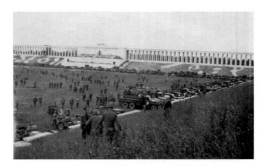

Former Nazi rallying grounds, Nuremberg, taken by Robby in the summer of 1945

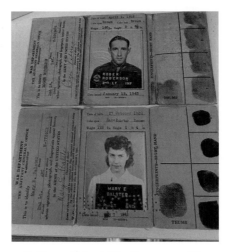

Robby and Mary's War Department IDs

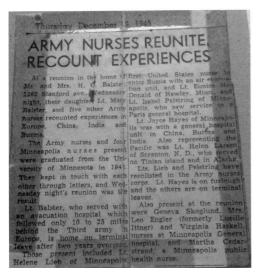

Newspaper article about the reunion Inga planned to entice Mary from her room, December 1945

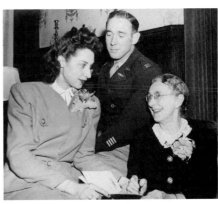

From left to right, Mary, "lovesick" Robby, and Gram

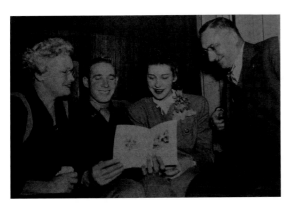

From left to right, Inga, Robby, Mary, and H. C. on the young couple's wedding day

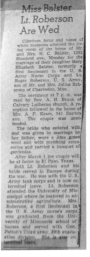

Newspaper announcement of Mary and Robby's wedding

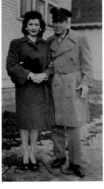

Mary and Robby leaving for honeymoon, 1946

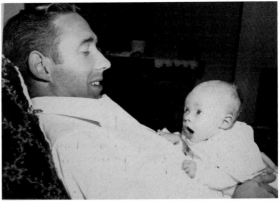

Robby with his and Mary's first baby, Madge Elizabeth

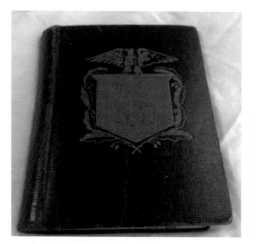

Mary's service diary

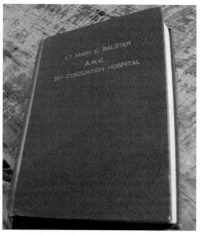

On Mary's 90th birthday, she gave this bound volume of letters to the author

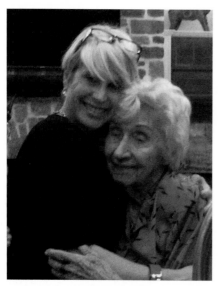

NCR Davis and her beloved mother, Mary at age 91

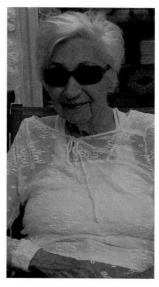

Mary at age 95, San Antonio, Texas

CHAPTER 16

On a Grassy Knoll near Sainte-Mère-Église

"To say aloud that he's handsome would be a wee bit redundant," Alabama was blathering on about Captain W. She and Mary sat on a grassy knoll. They were waiting for the hospital to be taken down. The unit was headed for Saint-Sauveur to take care of patients arriving from battles in and around Avranches.

Mary responded with only a slight agreement, saying that she supposed he was good-looking but that she hadn't really looked at him in that way, probably because of the age difference. And she never had been too enamored with men who "behaved so darn debonaire" because, in her book, they always turned out to be overly conceited. Nothing was more annoying and unappealing.

Since her response to Alabama was rooted in her original opinion about W, she considered the deceit a small one. And, universally speaking, she always feared men who seemed overly refined. She was convinced that they were secretly criticizing her, which, in turn, made her feel awkward, so she avoided the type. At first, she'd felt that W was no exception when she met him in Altrincham. She was sure that he analyzed her every action and, as a result, she'd get nervous and clumsy around him. She'd noticed his allure, the classic speech patterns, that elegance that commanded his movements. Those divine looks, "so blond and blue," she'd said, referring to his hair and eyes. His forehead was high, which Inga always had said was a sign of superior intellect. The distance between his cheekbones and chin was geometrically appealing, and his eyes were set wide, which she felt was more attractive than the typical Americans' more narrowly set eyes, like hers. Even though he'd appeared in the wards countless times, the women still swooned.

In her service diary she thumbed the pages to find the words she'd written about Robby; the only shave tail she'd ever met "without a line." Could W be the second suitor worthy of this compliment? Well, third, if she forced herself to count as far back as Zim. She remembered the guilt she'd undergone for comparing Robby to Zim. Now she was constantly swallowing guilt for comparing W to Robby, which seemed especially wrong. After all, W had been born into a privileged life. And even if he hadn't been born into wealth, he'd still had a lot more time to cultivate subtleties. W was already 40. Robby would only be 27 the following April.

Now she wished that her first impressions about W had been right. Her view of him had undergone a complete reversal since that lunch when Col. Bracher and Major Scanlon had introduced her and Mona to him. Since then, he'd shown her a side that was charitable, a man completely devoid of fulsomeness; there was nothing flamboyant about him. There was just an unbridled decency.

The reversal had begun in late spring. W had been the one to notice how emotionally wrecked she was when they were packing supplies headed to the Continent. She was in that rough patch. Now it seemed so ridiculously stupid to have been so weepy and whiny over having gotten kicked out of the Buckley billet and consequently having that massive fight with Mona. These days now? In Normandy? Why, she'd never think about crying over such inconsequential events. Nevertheless, it was W who had been the one to notice how upset she was at the time. He'd seen the tears plopping onto the necks of the blood bottles she was packing, so he'd grabbed her elbow, said it was time she took a break.

She'd followed him outside the supply tent, and they shared a couple of Lucky Strikes while she explained that it had been a trying week, month really. She hadn't heard from Robby in a while. And she and Mona weren't speaking to each other. She didn't care to go into the details with W but suffice it to say that the combination of several unfortunate events having taken place over just a few days had caused her to lose the ability to pack those darn blood bottles without losing her self-control. He said little, but his affect bore out an understated tenderness. There was an inherent acceptance and compassion for her circumstances but a quiet demeanor that suggested to her an assuredness that "this too shall pass."

On that day, England had restored itself to its typical soggy spring after months of drought, and cloud coverage offered an afternoon light that produced a translucence in their faces. She recalled his taking short drags on the cigarette he shared with her to make it last longer since she was taking such long drags. She also remembered that her voice quivered and sank under the heavy wet breeze, and she recalled how patient W had been. He would tap her hand as a signal that he didn't hear the last thing she'd whimpered,

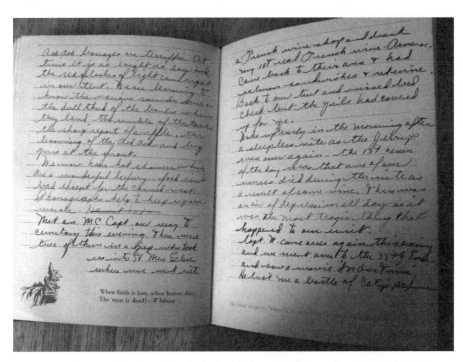

Mary's service diary mentioning the death of a nurse of the 39th, and Captain W

so she'd force herself to repeat the detail and then worry that she was offering too many details that this doctor surely didn't really care to know. But he was kind to put up with her droning.

She'd become a lot more like him since then, that is, from a clinical point of view. She'd learned that a good caregiver recognizes that the details of a patient's condition or injury are correlated with the patient's emotional needs. Often a patient needed the doctor to listen to what happened to him and his company in a battle, or he needed a nurse to hold his hand until he could fall asleep. The minute details of his needs were important to recognize and could greatly affect the patient's outcome. How that patient was handled emotionally was an important component of the healing process. She'd observed that this dynamic must be appreciated and understood by the doctor and the nurse, even when the army seemed to be much more interested in just getting the soldier back to the fighting, regardless of his emotional injuries.

W listened to her as he would have any patient. And because he'd handled her in this way, a trust in him began to form. Previously, when she'd sought Mona's or Alabama's counsel, their reactions had been similar. When it came to Mary's specific entanglements with beaus, Alabama never corrupted her listening with unwanted motherly advice or judgment. And Mona had stopped the practice altogether, too, so Mary became devoted to both and trusted them wholeheartedly.

Until today, Mary hadn't recalled the crying over the blood bottles and W's subsequent insistence that he take her somewhere to talk. Alabama's comment about W stirred her thoughts about all the people who'd become vitally important to her maintaining a satisfactory level of emotional health, enough to keep her afloat these days. Only two days ago, Mona told Mary that she'd come to accept her beguiling nature. She knew it was not going to change and was, in fact, that aspect of her personality that everyone found to be endearing.

Mona added that she'd decided to join the ranks of so many who were devoted to Mary and would love her despite her mild pitfalls or major insurrections. She said that the entire lot of Mary's admirers would just have to hope that any fallout from her choices wouldn't result in a dishonorable discharge or worse for her and anyone else caught in her fray.

CHAPTER 17

Lost Cots and Litters in the Sun

Since most of the 77 patients admitted to the unit's first day in Saint-Sauveur were German, Mary's fluency was crucial, especially during triage. She took every opportunity to help medics learn a few key German phrases. The EMs been issued translation cards, but if Mary was close by, it was easier to just ask her, as their hands were busy applying pressure from bleeding wounds, or wrapping tourniquets, or lifting patients from gurneys onto surgical tables. That night she forced herself to rest and write a quick update for her parents:

> August 1, 1944
> Dear Mom and Dad,
>   Am very tired and as soon as I finish this am going to write to Robby and hit this GI cot even though it's only 8 P.M. You know in the army you either work like the devil or you just sit. It's really a hard life to get used to and sometimes you're just exhausted but always get to rest. Of course in this type of unit it's not always that way. Half the time don't know where you're going to sleep the next nite but we're not particular if we have a bed anymore, for just the chance to lie down is enough. Someday I will tell you all about it—that is except for the things I'll never talk about.
>   Have some more requests and hope they get here before the war is over. Our mail has a hard time keeping up with us. Please send more Kleenex, Palmolive soap, clothespins, bobby pins, Eliz. Arden dusting powder, a couple of wash cloths and two tubes of M.F. [Max Factor] medium lipstick as Mona would like some. Am sending a money order as soon as we get paid and you can use what you need to cover the above and save the rest for me, please. Must close for now so until later Au Revoir and all my love,
>   Mary

When Mary reflected on those summer days in Normandy, she said that her unit collectively grew a resilience, a toughness to the conditions, and that taking care of the boys provided the incentive to overcome any brief wishes for self-comfort:

August 4, 1944
Dearest Family,

Sorry I have to write V Mail but have no other paper and still less time these days. Just got off duty and haven't stopped for 13 straight hours. It's work hard, eat like a horse, and sleep like a log these days. Too tired to be scared of bombs or anything else now. Feel wonderful and the boys tell me I don't have to roll out the pills or use the needle just to look at a picture of health and vitality is enough to make them well. Gee. They're wonderful patients and it's easy to see why we are winning this war. There's never a dull moment and it's all so interesting wouldn't trade it for anything. No time for recreation these days but spirits keep high because my honey writes every day. His letters begin "My Darling Wife" and are so darned sweet. To be able to see him just for 5 minutes would be all I would ask now but maybe it won't be too long now. Have so many interesting things to tell you after the war—they'll just have to wait until then. It's a wonderful feeling to really be doing my part at last and the time is going very fast. Write soon and often, please.

Lovingly,
Mary

On the morning of August 8, 1944, the unit's first day in Vitre, Poncho gingerly descended a golden slope of wheat stalks, balancing a silver tray that he'd picked up from God-alone-knew-where. Possibly he'd found it in a burned-out house in Saint-Sauveur. He and Mary were determined to establish themselves as the lead pilferers of the 39th, their collection of abandoned relics already beginning to rival the contents of an auction house. On the tray, four tin cups rolled about. He toted a bottle of champagne under each arm. At the bottom of the hill, Mary, Alabama, and Mona were amused at the sight of his trundling. There was a great deal of speculation as to what Poncho was "up to." When he got close enough for them to see his wares, Alabama teased him, asked if he'd left his maître d' uniform at the dry cleaners.

They needed to chuckle, as there had been a scare during convoy to Vitre the night before. Bombs had demolished a patch of the road, so the engineers and enlisted men had been forced to repair it just enough for the ambulances, supply trucks, and jeeps to pass over what Poncho described as "SNAFU."

Chief Maxson had figured that the nursing staff would be frightened about the halt, so Poncho had been sent around to each ambulance to explain the reason for the stop. He also informed the nurses that they didn't have to worry about being "sitting ducks," because right outside the 80th and 30th Divisions were guarding them, thanks to orders from General Patton.

Finally, the convoy had been able to complete the 104-mile trek and dumped them at Vitre by four that morning. They napped on the ground during the pre-dawn hours. When they woke to reveille and a can of rations, daylight revealed that they hadn't slept alone. Various unidentifiable bugs, some of them large enough to rival the size of small rodents, had been their sleeping companions. While they waited for the boys to finish the evac set-up, everywhere one could hear the billowy swishes of blankets being tossed about. Some of the insects inhabiting the blankets proved challenging to remove, their spindly, stubborn legs sticking to the olive drab woolens. The scene reminded Mary of "July, a year ago," when she and Mona had been covered in those black flies. Since Alabama hadn't been assigned to the 39th until the month after, she'd missed the black fly experience.

Alabama repeated what she'd said earlier that morning—that she didn't like the bugs one bit but that they paled in comparison to her need for one long gulp of safe drinking-water from Tennessee. She'd been the most vocal about the dirty French water that had to be "boiled to hell and back" before it was deemed safe enough to drink.

Poncho then proceeded to pop the cork from a Bollinger bottle and quipped, "What, Lt. O'Reilly, you don't like my water replacement?"

Poncho had been with the unit since last October when they were still in Tennessee. Mary often gave him her liquor rations after he'd volunteered many times to help her dig a fox hole. He often teased her since Robby had become a part of her life, saying that he guessed that her liquor rations must be going her "First Lieutenant's way" because she hadn't been sharing any with him lately. Poncho and Mary formed a strong bond, and even though familiarity with enlisted men was discouraged by the army, the realization was that when human beings are working together in horrific living conditions in a war zone attempting to save soldiers' lives, only a few superior officers successfully achieved a guarded distance between themselves and enlisted personnel.

In those early days of service on the Continent, rumors about the camp flew well above the average amount of chatter, most of it involving bets as to how fast the Allies would be able to liberate all of France. There had also been a lot of gossip about General Patton, many speculating that things might run a little differently once he became Commander of the Third Army. Officially, that day occurred on August 1, 1944, when the 39th was still in Saint-Sauveur, but Poncho's plans to celebrate the occasion with his three favorite lieutenants had to be postponed until Vitre. The patient load at Saint-Sauvuer had taken priority. August 2 and 3 had been the bloodiest days the unit had seen to date, their admission number hitting 125 on August 2, the highest they'd ever recorded. At the time, 125 admissions had seemed very challenging. Soon they would consider such a number to be a "light day."

Poncho raised a tin cup, apologizing for the delay in his having to put off his little toast. The gals followed suit. He added another tidbit. August 1 had also marked the 39th's six-month anniversary of foreign service.

The unit wasn't slammed with patients that morning, but based on news coming from the CZ (Communications Zone), they were expecting a large number of admissions later in the day. Poncho was hoping to get more accurate information as the day wore on, but he knew this might be the only time to share a brief toast. Afterwards, everyone hurried off to either write letters or catch up on laundry. It was Mary's intention to grab some sunlight and do some catching up on her sewing project that she'd begun with parachute scraps. Poncho joined her for a few minutes, scrambling about, helping her find more of the blue, green and orange pieces. She told him that she wanted to finish sewing a halter top for her friend Brownie and that Sgt. Jocus wanted something made for his wife. She spotted a less "buggy" knoll to spread out a blanket, and Poncho helped her lay out all the colored pieces of parachute fabric. As she tried to force herself to make final decisions about patterns, Poncho excused himself to get back to Chief Maxson's office tent. He was sure she'd have a list of tasks ready to dole out.

Alabama had been assigned night shift, too, so she pushed some of the parachute pieces off a corner of the blanket to create a spot to join Mary. When Alabama began to needle point, Mary asked her if she'd ever noticed that, in the army, "you either work like the devil or just sit."

Of course, she'd noticed, but the main thing on her mind while they were just sittin' was if Mary happened to know the whereabouts of the "bug powda."

But before Mary had a chance to think about where the bug powder could have hidden itself, Chief Maxson approached them. Naturally, they threw down their sewing and stood up to salute her.

She never minced words and proceeded to warn Mary that she needed to forget about those parachute scraps for the remainder of that day. She would be ordering Poncho to deliver a stack of towels that Mary would be sewing into washcloths, as the unit was in dire need.

Maxson never looked at Alabama. Obviously, this order was meant for Mary only.

Mary responded with a "yes, ma'am," but it seemed that she couldn't stop herself from following up the "yes ma'am" with a question. She wanted to know if her superior officer knew whether the sewing machine had made it in once piece after all the bumpy roads they'd traveled over the night before.

Alabama's eyebrows raised. She swallowed awfully hard. What the hell was Mary thinking asking the battleax that. Jesus, Mary was bold but dumb sometimes.

The assignment instantly doubled. Now Mary would be required to make *100* wash cloths sans sewing machine and have them finished *before* Lt. Balster reported for duty at 1500 hours.

Soon after, Mona entered the tent in time to find Mary cutting off the top of a new can of insect powder and pouring it into her sleeping bag. Clouds of white powder filled the tent, causing Mona and the bug exterminator to cough, gag, and then bail.

Now Mona figured out why they'd been having so many headaches. They weren't from chronic dehydration. They were from inhaling all that damn bug poison.

Mary pulled up her pants leg.

Mona gasped.

"What are those bites?"

Neither nurse could figure out what bug had caused the bites that covered Mary's legs. She looked like a leper. For various reasons they'd learned in nursing school, they knew it couldn't be any form of leprosy, and she certainly didn't have any loss of feeling where the rashes were, as she had scratched the hell out of those areas. No. They had to have been caused by some insect. The conversation became wildly speculative. They even wondered if naval ships from the Mediterranean had carried sand fly eggs to the Continent and now maybe they were in Normandy and had set up camp under Mary's skin.

To Mary, they sure felt like sand fly bites, the itching driving her just a little insane.

Mona didn't see how Mary with her present state of exhaustion combined with her itching misery was ever going to complete the washcloth assignment and get ready in time for 3:00 p.m. duty. She took over and quickly designed a towel template, laying out five towels, one on top of the other. They could cut the five towels into three strips of equal width and then cut five horizontal strips of equal size across the three strips. That was a total of 75. Before Mary knew it, they'd finished 105 cloths. Mary thought back to the letter she'd recently sent to her parents. She and Mona laughed at the irony of her asking Inga to send washcloths.

When Poncho delivered the towels, he'd reported back that they were now getting messages that casualties were going to be very bad by mid-afternoon.

Although General Patton had ordered the majority of the Third Army to make a direct march toward Paris, he'd assigned men from the 83rd Division (three regiments), the 121st Infantry (8th Division), and the 1st and

3rd Battalions of the 331st Infantry to move through Brittany. Their mission was to take the coastal towns of St. Malo and Dinard.

The few men ordered to take St. Malo and Dinard (often called the "hornets' nest" of Nazi power) fought through ponds, swamps, minefields, mortar, and artillery fire. Stone and concrete pillboxes too numerous to count littered the countryside, hiding machine guns that cross-fired to hold back Third Army troops who attempted to drive through double rows of steel gates.[1]

As a result, casualties were heavy. By the time Mary arrived for duty that afternoon, her patients were lined up on litters outside the hospital tents. Somehow, the unit had lost her cots. She couldn't believe it. The absolute morons. How could they lose cots?

During triage, her agitation increased. Soon, a sergeant found her in tears. Her boys were bleeding and baking in the sun.

They were trying to locate the cots. Also, someone was on his way to borrow some from the 6th Convalescent.

She counted. They would need at least 40 cots. She ordered him to find some PFCs, corporals, anyone to help shade the patients with anything they could muster—surgical drapes, or tarps, towels, anything. The boys didn't need to die of dehydration or heat stroke because some idiot lost the cots. They didn't have enough surgeons *or* cots to take care of all the boys.

She hurried inside the tent to wipe her face and blow her nose with her last Kleenex tissue. A pang of guilt overcame her for screaming at the sergeant, but she quickly regained her composure and ran back outside. There was no time for guilt.

By midnight the 39th admitted almost 500 patients. As horrific as that day was, there had been a silver lining. Earlier, the unit had captured a German captain, a surgeon no less, and four German medics. The doctor turned out to be a fine surgeon and helped the other surgeons of the 39th perform 124 surgeries that single August day, a record.

The two German medics who helped Mary in her ward that afternoon and evening were well trained, and once Mary had her 42 patients assessed, she ordered them to check on three critical prisoners of war while she wrote her report. The next day the three would be moved to their own tent if enough cots could be located so that the Allied wounded would not have to lie next to the enemy.

---

1   "Brothers-In-Arms: 83rd Division, 331st Infantry." Website Contributor Dave Curry in memory of his father Thomas Curry, 1999. Web. March 9, 2016. http://kb8tt.net/brothers/

CHAPTER 18

It's Just the Little Things, Daddy

There were three of them stuffed on one side, three on the other. A corporal had modified the ambulance to accommodate six nurses in preparation for the ride from Vitre to Arrou. At just past midnight, Mary, Mona, and Alabama crawled into the left-half of the ambulance and busily fiddled with their olive-drab blankets again, shaking their heads at the realization that in less than four weeks they'd become adept at nest-making, whether it was on the ground, in a slit trench, or in the back of an ambulance.

Their subconscious minds did a decent job of burying most of the memories of their time in Vitre. All that seemed to be left were blurred images and muted sounds that took over when they tried to fall asleep in the ambulance. Nobody wanted to talk about their individual patient care experiences.

Since Mary assumed that Robby was still a platoon leader, the burn cases associated with destroyed Sherman tanks haunted her.

> Daddy, I wish I could tell you each and every one of the past month's experiences—they're something I'll never forget and wouldn't have missed for the world and yet some of the events have been so awful I hope that I can forget them. It's funny, you know, I never used to have nightmares but guess it must be from some of the first days and nights when everything was so frightening. The boys have awful ones and we all just want to put our arms around them and tell them that they are safe. Golly my heart just aches for them, but a smile, a wisecrack, a bath, a backrub or just a talk with them is all they want.
>
> Today one of my eighteen-year-olds wanted to write a letter so, after I dug up the equipment for him to write with he said, "Mary, now you've got me all set up to write, and I can't think of a darn thing to say. I guess I'm just stupid—why I could write volumes about you and the Army Nurse Corps in just what I've seen and had done for me in the past two days."
>
> It's just little things like that, Daddy, that make all this hell much lighter. If we come back looking like a bunch of worn-out old women who no one will ever want after this war is past, well we will always have the satisfaction that we've really done our part and there are boys who will never forget. I don't complain about a thing after I see and hear what they've gone through for all of you back home and for us here.

In my daily work I make lots of decisions, everything from deciding when to give plasma, blood, etc., to dressing wounds. It's always, "Ask Mary," or "ask the nurse." It's a wonderful feeling to be able to go ahead on my own and know people have confidence in me. I get awfully lonesome for all of you but hope that when I do see you again, I'll be somewhat the same Mary that you last saw.

The boys think it's wonderful that we're right here with them, and I think we're privileged to be here and get a first opportunity to treat their wounds. But if it weren't for our aid men who are right on the firing line and give first aid all the while being shot at themselves, why we wouldn't be able to save half as many lives. Those guys do a beautiful job and in the hundreds of wounds I've dressed I've only found two infected ones and all the credit goes to those boys as they dump that sulfa powder into every wound and dress them, so they don't hemorrhage to death. All of our wounded say that they will never call a medic a "pill roller" again. The medics are at last getting the credit they deserve.

Every time we admit a young boy from a tank outfit, and he's messed up so badly and when other boys tell such awful tales it just gets to me, and all I can think of is that Rebel I love so much. He's not in the same army as I am, and I won't say which army he's in, but tanks, Daddy, the injuries are so terrible. I can't think of it and pray so hard every waking minute. If something happens to Robby, I'll just be a gypsy, that's all. There's no man who comes close to that sweet, beautiful, brown-eyed boy of mine. But Robby doesn't want me thinking or writing anything negative to you and the rest of the family. He says in all his letters to me that it's very important to remain positive and keep my chin up and all will turn out all right.

Gee the patients try to give us everything they have. Today I collected four chocolate bars, a lovely silk Jerry hanky that I'm saving for you, two cans of cheese, two sponges (little facial ones) and tomorrow one of our truck drivers is bringing Mona and me some fresh tomatoes… and our patients give us bullets and knives… We have so much stuff but lose at least half of it…

Well, Daddy, this is a jumbled letter, but having been a soldier yourself I know you understand. Boy, I know now what a good outfit you served with—the PFCs take the worst beating but where would we be without them?

Allow Mom to read this letter only if you think it won't worry her.

Lovingly,

Your GI girl, Mary

Months after Vitre, in early 1945, someone from the unit had been awarded leave to Paris. He brought back developed photographs of the 39th's early days in Normandy and left a stack of the photos in the Red Cross tent for everyone to look at during their breaks. There was one of Mona among them. Somebody made a comment that Mona's dimples were gone in the photograph.

They weren't really gone, Alabama had replied. It was a simple case of Mona not being able to stir up a smile at all during those days.

At some point during the ride to Arrou, Mary reached for Mona's hand. Mona held on tightly, then squirmed and murmured. Soon, she gave up efforts to hold back.

At first, Alabama didn't know who was crying. The ambulance bay was so dark.

Mary fuddled around with her free hand in search of Kleenex. Then she remembered that she'd used the last one back in Vitre. Finally, she found a piece of parachute fabric in the Val-Pack that she had borrowed from Mona. She'd inadvertently stored her Val-Pack in a box stuck in England. There couldn't have been a sorrier excuse for a tissue than parachute material, but it would have to suffice to help Mona dry her face and blow her nose.

She felt for a canteen and asked Mona to try to sit up a bit and take a few sips. Mona's cheeks were hot, despite the cold interior of the ambulance. It couldn't have been above 50 degrees Fahrenheit.

Alabama remained quiet. Not one interruption. Not one offer to help. Not a peep.

Once Mona was able to talk without sobbing, Mary encouraged her. She said it would help make it go away, whatever was bothering her so.

Nine days earlier Mona was the acting head nurse in Surgery. A patient had been admitted with multiple landmine wounds. He and a few others in his company had cut through an open field on foot to gain ground on a few enemy soldiers they'd spotted. When the mines exploded, some men fell instantly, but this patient apparently made it to a barn despite severe injuries.

By the time the EMs came across the carnage in the field, most had perished, but one of the medics thought to check a barn nearby. They found him there unconscious but still breathing. Mona had been occupied with triage, but when there was a lull in acute admissions she was to assist as needed. By the time she was able to help, the surgeon had already performed traumatic amputation of the left leg at the greater trochanter. To save the right leg, he debrided necrotic tissue that was embedded with manure. He didn't stop debriding until he hit the femur. But four days later, the surgeon had to take the leg after all because it wouldn't heal. There was speculation as to why he hadn't amputated it the first night. Mona knew why he hadn't. She'd overheard him. The surgeon couldn't look another boy in the eye after he'd been responsible for carving him into a double amputee.

The patient hung on for eight days. He was so brave, but sepsis overwhelmed him and by the time his death was imminent, he accepted his fate and expired holding Mona's hand that morning when most of the unit was packing for Arrou.

For the remainder of the ambulance ride, it wasn't necessary for anyone to talk about anything. Mona slept, her head nestled under Mary's arm.

A few days into their stint in Arrou, Mary and Mona had wondered why Alabama seemed so stoic during that ambulance ride. It was so uncharacteristic of her. And they knew it wasn't as if Alabama hadn't been suffering from her own grief at losing so many patients. She was extremely loving and held deep sympathy for her patients and her peers. Her lack of emotional display that night in the ambulance was simply a defense mechanism. During times of sheer agony, all of them, Mary said, sometimes resorted to habits formed during their youth. In Alabama's case, she fell back into that "good ole Southern denial" that aristocratics clung to when grief felt too much to bear.

Young ladies from Mountain Brook, Alabama, were reared to handle grief and loss privately. All the venues associated with death were to be viewed as dignified social gatherings. Any display of grief, then, was forbidden in the open, and the death of a friend was looked at as a responsibility in which one took food, wine, and beer to the grieving family.

If the death occurred in someone's own family, crying was considered weak and never done in public. Any display of grief was to be done in the privacy of one's home just after a loved one died. Emotional outbursts and excessive blubbering were expected to be completed within a few hours of losing the loved one. Then all efforts turned to drying the tears and powdering the swollen face before any planned events were to take place: the wake; the funeral, which was held at the church, synagogue, or funeral home; the cemetery; the dead person's family home. Death had to be accepted. But it had to be handled with decorum and a stiff upper lip. Emotional "hurling" of any kind in front of friends, peers, and business associates topped the "DO NOT" list of the implied etiquette guide for living and dying in the South. All children from "good families" in Mountain Brook knew these things by their sixth birthday, and God help them if they didn't abide by these expectations because a "whippin'" (spanking) would be waiting for the child once back at the homestead.

When Alabama's father's brother was dying, he told Elizabeth that he wanted to go to her uncle's home to sit with "Bubba" until he passed on. Many southerners refer to their sons and brothers as "Bubba." It's a term of endearment.

A few hours later, her uncle passed away. The funeral director (undertaker) arrived and whispered to his boys to place Mr. O'Reilly's body on the stretcher. Alabama's father got up, followed the young men through the home and toward the front door. When they reached the foyer, her father became overwhelmed. He hadn't shed one tear of grief over losing Bubba, the man who'd always been his best friend, this person whom he loved as much as God, Jesus, his wife, and his daughter Elizabeth. No. He had not cried, screamed, or bawled.

Instead, just as the undertaker opened the front doors of his brother's home, the shock of sunlight carried with it an implication that life was still going on outside. Just after having pushed the double front doors back against the walls as wide as they would go to make room for the stretcher's exit, he looked over at Mr. O'Reilly and noticed he was turning pale. But before the undertaker could get around his boys and the stretcher that carried Alabama's dead uncle, her father hit the marble floor hard, flat on his back.

Early on, then, Alabama had observed that when the soul refuses to outwardly grieve, the mind has one recourse—it will force the body to check out, some way, somehow, to emotionally accept the unacceptable. Crying—not permissible. Talking about death—never. Fainting—understandable but not recommended.

This "chin-up" approach was not unlike the cultural norms that shaped Mary's rearing in the mid-west, although Mary's also held to a fatalism when she forced herself to face the present.

> … The darn Jerrys have been doing a lot of strafing and either don't know a hospital at nite or don't give a darn, but a couple of our sister evacs have gotten it—blackout is difficult with a tent setup you know, and they say they can't see the Red Crosses from up there. Oh, well, if we get it, we do, that's all… Don't tell Mom this but you've no doubt seen it in the papers anyway. Last nite when they were flying low a Lt. in my ward who was over here last war and treated me just like you would, anyway he had a cot with a pile of blankets for me to crawl under if they started anything, but I wouldn't have left my boy last nite if a thousand Jerrys came over. I don't know but… when you're on duty you never think of being scared.

The newly liberated French towns along the southern flanks of Patton's Third showed their appreciation to their new Allied occupiers in the form of bartering. Fresh fruit had been a luxury for months, but once they had settled in at Arrou, finally Mona and Mary escaped the 39th long enough to barter candy and cigarettes for fresh apples and a few eggs. They reached their living quarters and saw that Alabama had also been successful at bartering, having traded a pound of coffee for a quart of champagne and secured three more fresh eggs for a bar of soap.

The tents were set up near a spectacular lake, the perfect place for providing fresh water for Mary to treat herself to a shampoo and, in the process, hopefully negate Chief Maxson's latest criticisms.

Chiefee had said "not to blame" her if she "ended up with bugs" in her hair, it was "so long" and that she "should ask Lt. O'Reilly [to] cut off four or five inches when they had a break in patient load." Oh yes, she would deny Chiefee the satisfaction of making one more snide comment about her hair. She'd change into the green halter she'd made for Brownie but hadn't had a chance to give her yet. It would be the perfect top to wear to the lake since the parachute material she'd made the halter from shed water so well. And she'd take her helmet to scoop up the fresh water from the lake's edge and treat herself to a shampoo—a rigorous one—just in case the old battleax was onto something and there *were* bugs crawling around.

Not three minutes later, Alabama and Mona heard a yelp and a splash.

Bees had been more than a nuisance since they had arrived at Arrou. Everyone had been stung numerous times, and Mary's right ring finger had swelled so much from a sting the day before that Mona thought she might be forced to take Mary to the OR and search for a tool to cut off her opal ring.

Just as she knelt at the water's edge, the bees swarmed, possibly interpreting Brownie's green halter as a flower. A startled Mary waved her helmet in front of her body, attempting to ward off the bees, but she lost her balance. Her body tipped forward. Just after a realization that there would be no regaining her balance, a staccato scream followed. She hit the lake full throttle, slapped the water's surface, and the bees swarmed away.

The first one to hear the scream was Alabama. At the water's edge, she found the bottle of Rayne Shampoo and tossed it in the water. Mary might as well go ahead and shampoo while she was in the lake.

Mary reported to duty that evening with clean hair, albeit quite damp, but decided that everyone would assume she had fallen victim to the rains that now blanketed the 39th.

At summer's end on the Western Front, saturating rains contributed to astounding trench foot statistics while booby traps and land mines emerged as the greatest threats to soldiers' lives—that is, if they survived the trip on the "litter" from the battlefield. Litters were makeshift gurneys that the EMs used to cart the soldiers back to wherever the closest evacuation hospital happened to be set up. Medics were to assess the soldier's injuries, apply tourniquets (but not so tightly, as they were learning from the nurses and physicians) and perform other first aid that was as patchwork as it gets. For that reason, General Patton insisted that the evacuation hospitals that supported his Third Army troops would set up their surgical and medical tents as close to the battles as possible. General Patton's plans didn't always pan out, evidenced by a letter Mary had written to her family when the unit was still in Arrou, dated August 16, 1944:

> You can tell by the news how scattered the front is. The other day one of the hospitals moved up and had to wait on the outskirts of a certain town while they finished up the street fighting. And sometimes you get in a spot where your own artillery is behind you. This sure is a crazy war and you probably won't believe some of my tall tales when I get home. Don't worry. I don't intend to tell you anything gruesome because no one wants to forget that part any faster than I do.

Ideally, the medic was to tag each patient with name, rank, serial number and list of injuries, but such an orderly and detailed list was not likely to happen during the throes of battle. Mary discovered this reality during the last night shift she worked before the 39th Evac left Arrou.

> Didn't get very far with this letter this a.m. 'cause my sickest patient who I held my breath for all nite decided to vomit a pile of blood, and I got right in the line of his fire. Gee. Last night I took his temp at 8 and it was 104, so I quick reported it, and they took him to surgery and removed a large piece of shrapnel which had lodged between the vertebrae. He sure was a sick boy only 19 and I stayed with him the rest of the nite and let the boys take care of the others…

During the last week of August, word around the 39th was that they would have to give up their lake view and head toward Nogent-sur-Seine. TUSA (Third United States Army) was attempting a rapid advance toward the Moselle River but became hampered by lack of gasoline. SHAEF (Supreme Headquarters Allied Expeditionary Force), run by the politically astute Eisenhower, had promised General Montgomery most of the gas supply, leaving little fuel for General Patton to achieve his goal to drive the Germans back persistently and rapidly to the Rhineland.

"To say that General Patton is PO'd [pissed off] would be the understatement of the century," Poncho muttered, as he began the mundane task of deconstructing the tents that had been erected only six days before. He rounded up the medical personnel. They had orders to pack and be ready to board the 6×6 trucks no later than 1800. Someone wanted to know why the medical personnel weren't traveling by ambulance this time. The answer was because their patients were either too wounded or too sick to return to the fighting and there was no relief evac expected to take over their care. The only choice was to take the patients with them in the ambulances.

The 39th had been compelled to borrow even more ambulances from the 109th and the 403rd Medical Collecting Company just to accommodate all the patients going with them to Nogent-sur-Seine.

By 1900, the 6×6s were lined up in the convoy. Eleven nurses piled in the 6×6 that included Mona, Alabama, Mary, Brownie, Chief Maxson, and others. W had stayed in Vitre to manage the patients who had been too sick to move but had written to Mary while he was away. The letters held a confession that he'd fallen in love with her. He caught up to the unit in time to catch the convoy leaving Arrou. Mona muttered, "Here he comes, like a bee to honey," when he stopped by the 6×6 to say hello to Mary.

Almost halfway to Nogent-sur-Seine, the passengers in the 6×6 entered what one of the passengers later referred to as "some sort of collapse of time." Just

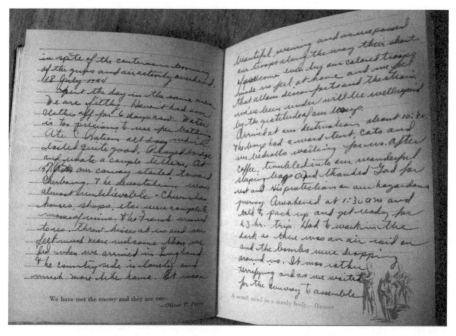

Mary's service diary document air raids and bombs

before 2220, high-pitched whistling followed by a long series of low-pitched rumbling made it difficult to distinguish mortar explosions from thunderclaps. Someone yelled, wondering if the sounds were from thunder or from bombs.

Before anyone could answer, a jolt of immense force hit the vehicle, a thrust so weighted and heavy that it propelled them from their seated positions, toppling and flipping their bodies around and out the back and sides of the 6×6.

CHAPTER 19

You Can't Blame These Boys

"Oh, yes, it was a white Christmas at home, and I had all my loved ones around me, including my Rebel. There was turkey for dinner and banana splits for dessert. I had on a beautiful red dress and high-heeled shoes and some very sheer silk stockings. And later I saw myself taking a bubble bath full of the hottest water ever, and then I crawled into some clean white sheets."

Dagny was at Mary's bedside and had been the charge nurse watching over her as a patient in the Medical Ward. She'd wanted to know what Mary had been dreaming—she seemed to have been humming something. It had been a Christmas dream, so Dagny said since the dream revealed turkey and banana splits, she would take it as a positive sign that Mary would be okay. There were two others lurking about, too—Poncho and Redmond, who simultaneously volunteered to run to the mess and grab as much chow as Mary wanted.

Mary wondered how long she could have been concussed. The last time she was "in the world," as she said, Redmond was convalescing but certainly not at a level of health that he could be running around the unit with Poncho. Dagny said that most of the unit agreed that Mary's condition upset Redmond so much that in two days' time he had willed himself to join the healthy ranks again just so that he could bring Mary back.

Dagny told her that Captain W had written an order that she was to spend one more night in the Medical Ward followed by one more day of tent rest before returning to shift duty.

September 3, 1944
Dearest Family,
    Guess I've neglected you the past week, but it really couldn't be helped. Have a couple hours off this afternoon. It's getting dark so early now can't hardly write after duty—just managed to get a few lines off to Robby but even had to neglect him for about 4 days. We moved again and had a smashup on the way. A weapons carrier hit the 6×6 that 11 of us nurses were riding in—no one was killed tho but just bruised up and I got a scalp laceration

and a lovely big bump on the head but am ok now so don't worry... Anyway, we're a bunch of grateful girls...

Our mail is lost again. Sgt. Parent was gone 2 days looking for it and came back with a few letters—all from the ETO, however, and at least I heard from Robby. He's been so darned faithful and guess I would go crazy if I didn't hear from him at least, but sure do miss those letters from home.

As our supply line gets longer everything is harder to get—gasoline is our biggest problem now.

It's been rainy and very cold the last couple days so am wearing long underwear already. Don't know what we'll do when winter comes but maybe we won't have to worry about that. Doubt seriously that I'll be home for Xmas and if the rumors are true, we'll probably be where it's nice and warm—all of our group won't but my age and length of service is against me. But maybe things will happen there, so we won't have to go after all.

Anyway, wish we'd get a short leave just to get away from it all, would do us a world of good. We have one girl who is on the verge of a nervous breakdown—guess her mom's not well and she says she cannot take it much longer. She was on maneuvers with us, and I sure feel sorry for her. It really isn't so bad except in the evenings when there's time to think of your loved ones and you miss everything so darn much but when on duty the time goes fast, and the boys appreciate us so. We do everything from nursing care to writing letters and mailing packages for them. They'd just rather talk than anything and tease us about everything from the way we put our leggings on in the dark every morning to the way our hair is combed. I swear they don't miss a thing but they're all wonderful boys and have the utmost respect for us.

Our own boys are as grand as ever and I swear if I asked one of them to jump in the river he would. They sure keep me busy fixing their clothes and now they turn their money over to me to send home for them before they gamble it or drink it away. I gave one of my 19 yr. old ward boys a lecture the other day because he has been getting hold of some rotten stuff to drink and just throwing his money away so yesterday after he got paid, he came to me with his whole salary and had me send it to his mom. He's really a good kid and you can't blame these boys for anything they do—gosh we can't go any place or do anything and it's pretty tough on some of the boys...

It's now evening, and duty is done for the day and after I write to Robby am going to bed. Sure would freeze if it wasn't for this sleeping bag. I just button it up and crawl in from the top and am as snug as a bug in a rug, but it is cold in the morning and so darn dark. We use our flashlites but have to be so careful about blackout they don't do much good. It sure will be wonderful to be able to turn a lite on and not have to worry about any light showing from the outside...

Private Redmond, Franz and Karl (the German prisoners of war who had turned into excellent ward boys), and two sentries kept Mary's shift that night tolerable. The 39th admitted 60 more soldiers, Mary's Medical Ward taking in 22. Chief Maxson put Mary as the charge nurse for night duty on the Medical Ward for the remainder of September, unless casualty numbers overwhelmed them and then she'd be asked to relieve nurses in Surgical.

Mary's ward consisted of seven transfers from the 109th Evac, five Americans and two Germans, all suffering from the usual—malaria, trench foot and

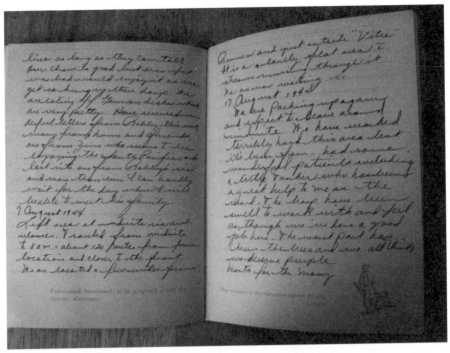

The "little tanker" is possibly Private Redmond

pneumonia. Then there were 22 more admissions to her ward that night, 20 of them German. Redmond was still helping her on the ward and asked her why she always got "stuck with all the Krauts." One of the prisoners of war was a 20-year-old who said that he was 17 when he was walking home from school one day in his little town in northern Germany. He and his friends got stopped by Gestapo and were ordered to get in the jeep. From there, they were taken to a military training camp and were enlisted in the German infantry. They were never allowed to go home to tell their parents goodbye. Mary had him as a patient convalescing after his right leg had been amputated but said that he still counted himself lucky. It was better to be a prisoner of war in an American hospital than it was to be a soldier in his own army.

Redmond wanted to know how he could help her on the shift that night. She needed hot water as fast as he could get it to her. She had five patients who needed their bandages changed, and maintaining a sterile environment wasn't easy.

So, he lit the little oil stove and heated two buckets full of water and began the trek back down the center aisle of the tent heading toward Mary.

She was taking the temperature of a post-operative patient that Redmond said was acting "crazier than a hoot owl" and wanted to know what was wrong with him. It was the sodium pentothal. The doctors were ordering it as an experiment. The latest clinical findings had said that keeping the patient in this state might allow the brain to heal. Redmond's job would be to remind Mary every 90 minutes to check that patient to see if the barbiturate was wearing off. Redmond said he'd be sure to do so because he didn't want the guy waking up the whole tent with "all that hollering."

The patient had been causing quite a racket for the last several minutes so there had been no telling how long Chief Maxson had been standing behind Mary and Redmond. Mary had thought Maxson was managing Surgical for the evening. With arms folded and a tucked chin, she asked Mary what *he* was doing there, which caused confusion since Mary couldn't understand why Chiefee would ask her why the patient was there. Then Maxson said that she didn't mean the *patient*. She was referring to the *private*—Redmond.

But before Mary had a chance to answer, Redmond said that he was going to just stick with Mary and help her until the army could find his tank outfit for him again, adding, "Mary's my girlfriend and I'm gonna do all I can for her and her patients."

Mary wrote to her sister Nancy the next morning, rehashing Redmond's explanation to Chief Maxson—"Gee, Nan, I thought I was going to faint from embarrassment."

CHAPTER 20

Got into a Little Dutch

Despite her devotion to Robby, Mary still held to the notion that her "R&R" time was an important component of her psychological wellbeing. Remaining "cooped up" with nothing to look forward to except another 12-hour shift of watching boys die and others suffer for days on end did not seem at all advisable.

W learned that the 39th would be moving from Nogent-sur-Seine soon. There'd been talk among the medical personnel that a few wonderful little French cafés had re-opened. He rounded up a couple more officers and secured two jeeps for a night away from chow and Red Cross popcorn and cookies. Mona was between beaus, so Mary talked her into going along. W arranged for her to date a distinctively handsome officer from a tank battalion. After meeting Major Bryson, both gals agreed that he was "just about as handsome as they come" and seemed to be "on the beam but definitely." Alabama volunteered to stay behind and pack Mona and Mary's belongings for the next day's trip to Vertus.

Two other nurses went along with their two officer dates in a second jeep. As Mary recalled, the restaurant was only about a mile and a half from the post. Pockets of Germans were still hiding in the hills, and snipers weren't all that uncommon, either so it was decided that Le Flaubert was their safest venue for the evening. The café had been ransacked by the Germans and had been closed for almost four years. The chef/owner held out for better days, and soon war-weary and hungry Allies became the first among many appreciative patrons who were in dire need of celebrating a return to normalcy.

The eight Americans entered the place sopping wet and sloshed about with muddy boots. The nurses wore their four-buckle overshoes that kept their feet warm and dry. They were led to a quaint back room with a marble fireplace.

A red cloth covered the dining table, and a sideboard was adorned with wine bottles of various shapes.

Soon, each of them left behind the horrific images they'd witnessed for weeks. For seven hours they drank champagne (GI tested-only), ate fresh trout caught from the Seine, and munched on baguettes that were still warm, having been freshly baked in a stone oven. Each couple shared a serving of crème brulée, still quite rare because of the hen and sugar shortage. W allowed Mary the entire dessert, as he had observed her weakness for sweets and said that she'd been so generous to share her Gram's mocha cakes every time she got a box from home.

At blackout, a waiter appeared and ceremoniously draped a black cloth over the single window. Someone asked him in French if it would be okay to light the fireplace that was in the back left corner of the quaint room. The waiter obliged, then apologized for the dim ambience, but he was certain that all Americans in the room understood the strict blackout conditions.

Mary was lost in thought. What was it about the place? There was something comforting in the little dining room. Then she remembered. The sideboard, the quaint ambience, everything about the room reminded her of that dessert table at the Hotel Jefferson, the one that had been decorated to resemble a French town. Everything felt comforting tonight because it reminded her of the last night she'd spent with Zim.

Such innocent times.

And now, she didn't even know where Zim was. Probably in the Pacific. Jesus Christ.

***

A distant rumbling brought her attention to the present. She prayed that Robby was in some place away from the horror.

Out loud, she wondered if they should be heading back.

Everyone agreed, and the nurses left the table to fetch their four-buckle overshoes since the rain had not let up. One of them speculated as to whether Vertus had any buildings left or if they'd be in tents again. Mona said that she'd heard Col. Bracher had sent an advance party and that no such luck would be had. No buildings worth fixing up were there. Tents it would be—again.

Mary struggled to get the left overshoe on. It just wouldn't go.

Mona sat in a dining chair opposite her. She grabbed Mary's left foot and propped it in her lap.

"Shit, it's full of edema," Mona said.

Did Mary recall injuring it? Maybe during the truck wreck? Maybe no one had noticed because all were so concerned about her concussion.

The foot was red, but it didn't look like gout to any of the nurses. Nor did it look like cellulitis. Both of those ailments would be very painful to the touch.

Mary confirmed that the foot didn't hurt, that it was just annoying because her shoe had begun to feel tight while they'd been eating. But since Mona had pulled it off to examine her foot, the swelling was now preventing her shoe from going back on, so she'd have to carry the shoe and just wear the four-buckle overshoe by itself.

***

When the blast hit, the staff were still serving a few locals in the main dining room. The front door of the enterprise blew open. A young French woman screamed.

In the smaller dining room, the force shattered the window, and the black drape was sucked right out, following the glass out into the open air. Everyone in the room, including the chef and waiter, hit the floor out of instinct. Mary and Mona crawled underneath the dining table. The other two nurses took cover under the sideboard.

Their eardrums popped, and the group began swallowing their saliva to try to equalize the pressure. The old wide-planked floor was christened with glass of all colors and shapes. There was hardly a safe, clean place on the floor for those lying flat to place their hands down to support their getting back up.

Smoke, thick and smothering, filled the room.

The waiter yelled, "Fire! Exit, Exit!"

The main dining room had burst into flames. There were more screams and hard crackling sounds. Everyone knew it would take only a few minutes before the entire restaurant became a tinder box.

Mona's date took over. They would make a crawling train by touching the shoes of the person ahead of them. Bryson and the waiter reached the blown-out window of the small room and pulled each guest out until the train of people was out of the building. W was the last out, having counted each person to make certain all had exited. The café continued to burn, and when the flames reached the kitchen, another explosion sounded like it had cracked open an entrance to hell.

"Probably hit a gas line," W muttered.

The flames were bright—uncomfortable for their eyes to look at for too long.

There was no way to put out the fire, but the waiter reassured the patrons that the buildings close to the restaurant were unoccupied. The Germans had driven out all the other enterprises. No business other than La Flaubert had re-established.

The rumbling sounded distant once again, so the eight members of the 39th decided to risk the ride back to camp.

***

When Mona and Mary reached their tent, Mona tripped on Mary's ammo box, waking Alabama. They apologized to her, but since she was awake, did Alabama know if they had missed Chiefee's bed check?

Not amused at having been woken, Alabama offered no more than a "no comment" and rolled over to face the tent wall and grab the sleepiness before it left her.

"Well, shit," Mona said, and she and Mary crawled into their sleeping bags fully clothed in their fatigues. No sense in changing attire. They would be rising to reveille and knew to expect a "knock-knock, hello" from Poncho soon, as they were all but certain Chiefee would send him to summon their presence.

Three hours later, Mary opened the flap and peeked out at him, then asked if the firing squad was ready. Poncho had an uncanny way of mixing concern with curiosity, so on the way to Chief Maxson's HQ, he wanted to know why they'd missed bed check.

On arrival at Lt. Maxson's tent Poncho announced that he had retrieved Lts. Balster and Ames. Maxson responded by asking for Lt. Balster first.

> When Chiefee called me to her office I put on my best military manners with a snappy salute and about face included. She said she was very surprised and was beginning to have high hopes for me because I was such an improvement from a year ago and all that slush. She just made me read the article of war dealing with AWOL and said that next time all of us would get a Court Martial. But the oldest girl in the group really caught it and is getting transferred. She called her a professional offender and really threw all the books at her. Don't tell Robby 'cause I just didn't mention it to him. He's pretty GI and as far as rules and regulations are concerned, he wants me to be too, and I must say I have been towing the mark, but it just isn't in me to be too good.

Mona's chastisement followed Mary's punishment. Although it was Mona's first infraction, her nerves completely overreacted when she overheard Mary reading the Articles of War regarding AWOL. She had to excuse herself to Poncho and head to the latrine. But her warm relationship with Maxson, combined with her stellar military record, held her in good stead, and all she got was a few months' delay in her promotion to first lieutenant. Her relief at having been handed less than a slap on the wrist gave her the confidence to explain to Maxson that Mary was ill and that she'd like her professional opinion about the swelling in Mary's foot.

The chief hadn't noticed Mary limping, but Mona assured her that Mary's inability to put on her left overshoe was partly to blame for their delay in returning to post the night before. Poncho was ordered to find Lt. Balster again. He didn't have to go far.

Mary was far more upset about Mona's potential punishment than she had been about her own. She was used to it, after all. Mona couldn't even have imagined getting into this predicament. Poncho found her pacing and smoking just a few tents south of Lt. Maxson's office. Everything was going to be fine, Poncho assured Mary, but Chief did ask for her to return to her office.

Chief Maxson ordered Mary to sit down and pull off her left boot, but Mary informed her and Mona that the swelling had moved to her right foot. A confused Mona and a skeptical Maxson suggested that she pull off both boots, then. Mona couldn't believe it. The edema had moved.

Chief Maxson asked a series of clinical questions—when had the swelling started, did Mary have an insect bite or a cut anywhere on either foot, had this happened before, etc.

Two days before, Mary had noticed swelling around the bottom of her right thumb but had attributed it to maybe a bee sting, but then the swelling moved to the left foot. But this morning, it moved to the right foot. Honestly, she was baffled.

Maxson agreed with the clinical assertion that the swelling wasn't the result of gout or cellulitis, but that, regardless of its cause, Mary was ordered to immediate bed rest until the swelling left. Maxson added more "slush," something along the lines that this was the first time in Mary's service in the unit in which she had not only taken responsibility for her penchant toward impulsivity and poor decisions but went so far as not to have offered this idiopathic swelling as an excuse.[1]

While Mary was relegated to bed rest, she wrote correspondence to Robby, Lorraine, her parents, and sister Nancy. Poncho stopped by her tent to check on her, and she asked him to take all her latest letters to Sgt. Parent to mail. In a letter to her father, she expressed her latest sentiments:

> ... Gosh, the news hasn't looked very good the last couple days and it's very rough at the front. My heart just aches for our boys and at times I just can't hold the tears back when they come in. Have acquired a bitter hatred for our enemy, and it's difficult to be kind to

---

1   Mary's mysterious condition was hereditary angioedema, not known in the 1940s.

them even when they're wounded and especially after hearing some of the tales our boys tell of their treatment in their hospitals before the French cities were liberated.

September 8, 1944
My dearest Family,

I'm half asleep but as I can't seem to really fall back guess I'll write some lines to you. Am on nite duty again and in about an hour nite nurses can take showers and would hate to sleep thru that especially today as we moved again and that always means sleeping in one's clothes for a couple of days…

Some of our boys came in late last nite so slept on my ward. As I had to stay on duty decided to lie down myself and had gotten sound asleep when there were some terrific barrages, and it was 4th of July again. Anyway, I woke up screaming for help, and then I was afraid that I woke the boys who weren't already awake with my shouting. The boys were swell though and came over to my bed and did their best to comfort me. After that I couldn't sleep so then was called to another ward to take over 'cause the nurse there got sick. Came back to my own ward and heated water for the boys to wash, and they sure appreciated it and were so cute. They gave me oranges and some sugar for it.

Am now on duty again and as the ambulances left a little while ago know I'm going to have a busy nite so will finish then and get one off to Robby before the fireworks start. It's chilly already and before morning it gets just awful. Gee, hate to think of the winter but think there will be some changes by that time. Have reconciled myself to the fact that it will be some time before we get home as there are so many others who have been overseas so much longer. Anyway, we'll probably get stuck with the Army of Occupation…

Just heard there's going to be a show tonite—a new film called "Christmas Holiday" so if I don't have any pts. by 9 am going to go. Last week they had "Going My Way" with Bing Crosby…

Mona is on nites too now so that makes us both happy. She's really the best friend a girl could have, and we stick by each other thru thick and thin. We sure have a bunch of swell girls and when the inspectors were here the other day from our Army's hdqs., they told the CO that they'd never seen as an attractive bunch of nurses in any group as here. We also received a letter from Hdq. [Headquarters] complementing us on our work here, our setup and a special complement to our mess officer…

Gee, that Kleenex came just in time 'cause I just was practically down to my reserve. Please keep sending Kleenex won't you. You didn't ask me what I'd like for Xmas yet but I'll tell you now so it will get here by the time I need it. For one thing I would like a new Fuller hairbrush and comb or are they impossible to get now? Also, some cosmetics, you know the usual brands—Merle Norman Med Powder, base, M.F. lipstick, Merle Norman crème rouge and some Coty L'Aimant powder. And, as I never lose my appetite, food is another request. Pabst-ett cheese, fruit cake, cookies, and candy.

Could also use some more notions, Mom, some white thread, safety pins and buttons. As Robby has been persistent to know what I want am going to tell him tonite too. I really hate to, but he said in his last letter he'd be angry if I didn't tell him. Gosh, if only I could see him—that's all I really want that and to get back home again is all I'll ever want now. It sure won't take much to satisfy me after this war if I only have my loved ones with me.

It's now the next evening and I really intend to finish this time. It gets so cold here at nite can hardly write. Most of my patients are in surgery now and am caught up with my work till they come back. I'd much rather be busy as the time goes fast and don't get as cold…

Well, here it is one a.m. and since I last sat down have been busy with patients returning from surgery and crazier than hoot owls as they give most of them pentothal which acts like liquor. Have all my hot water bottles in use and most of my blankets and they're still shivering. As for myself have on long underwear, overshoes, and a wool OD shirt, my wool slacks because it's Sunday, sweater and my combat suit which is just like a ski suit—thank goodness for my long hair which about touches my shoulders now and keeps me warm. The boys love it this way, but Chiefee doesn't. My helmet is too heavy to wear all the time and besides it isn't warm, so I only put it on when there's a lot of akak in case of flak...

Just sewed my new shoulder insignia on—they're rather pretty but for obvious reasons can't describe them. Have some of the boys' to sew on and some more stripes, but my hands are too cold to sew now.

Slept from 8 a.m.—5 p.m. yesterday so am not sleepy tonight. I usually fill my canteen with boiling water, and it sure keeps my feet nice and warm when I go to bed. Have 4 blankets, my sleeping bag, and a comforter and use them all. I swear I don't know how our poor boys can stand it sleeping in fox holes. They come in chilled to the bone and then I think how lucky we are here.

Bought some things in a town the other day and will send them home as soon as I get Gram something so I can send them all in one box. Guess they'll be your Xmas presents now 'cause they won't get there much before I don't imagine. As we don't get full value for our money here intend to change most of it into American currency and send it home from now on.

Have some medications to give so will finish this off now and hope I'll get lots of letters from all of you at mail call tomorrow.

All my love,
Mary

Third Army pressed on, liberating French towns during the fall of 1944. Many times, it was rumored that General Patton's proximity was very close to the 39th Evac. His famous advance against Nancy left a massive casualty count in its wake. September 9, 1944, became known as "Blood Day" for TUSA. Third Army liberated Nancy by September 15, but the 39th admitted over 450 critically wounded patients during those six days. The 460th Motor Ambulance Company was ordered to evacuate any wounded who were able to travel via ambulance or other motor means to relieve the now completely overwhelmed 39th.

September 19, 1944
Dearest Daddy:
It's 3 o'clock in the morning which makes 8 down and 4 to go. Hours of duty I mean...
Casualties have been severe and heavy and so we've all been double timing it. After 7 a.m. am so tired just fall into bed and we don't come to until 5 p.m. which leaves 2 hrs. out of the 24 to take a shower, eat, and do laundry, so you can see why I haven't had time to write. We are hoping for a break soon, but we just can't take one as long as our boys need us and I'm sure no one wants to. Everyone is irritable and tense. Gosh, sometimes I think I can't look at one more wound or some awful sight. Tonite the tears came to my eyes when we admitted a poor boy who was shot down last May and has been a prisoner until the town

in which he was held was liberated by our soldiers. Within 6 hrs. after our troops moved in, they had those boys here and when they brought him in, I shivered. An amputated arm, part of his nose gone, can't close his mouth and a horribly scarred face from gasoline burns from his plane. His eyes and head are bandaged but when I spoke to him as he was brought in, he said, "My God an American girl—I want to cry." And he did, and he didn't know it, but I did too. And that's just one in the hundreds that are brought in. And then there's the shell shock cause (we call it combat exhaustion) they're really pitiful but respond well to the treatment they are given in this war.

We keep saying it just can't go on much longer. We really don't know much about the news except from our pts., it's impossible to keep track of the days and all we care about is our work, eat and sleep. Our mess is super. I think our mess officer deserves a gold star because mess means so much, as it's the only time we really relax. The mess tent is fixed up cute now—have long tables covered with oil cloth, wicker chairs, lovely colored dishes, and nice silver. Most of it is confiscated material but as they didn't have time to take it with them, we use it—besides, think we're feeding half the German army now. Also have a radio in the mess hall which is always tuned in to the best music. Conversation is shop talk and what we're going to do when we get home.

It's been raining and so is terribly muddy. We have to observe such strict blackout it's really rough at nite getting around but as there's still air activity no one breaks blackout regulations. Remember that PFC I used to talk about on maneuvers? Well, he's a corporal now and is up for a Sgt's rating. They've finally recognized his ability—he's better than an E.M.—at least better than many I've seen. Anyway, he takes me to midnite chow every nite. We're not supposed to go around in the blackout alone at nite so he told the nurse on his ward that he was going to take me to supper every nite. As she's one of my best friends never a word is said but then there's no harm in it that I can see, but as you know the army sees things differently—especially the 39th, but what they don't know won't hurt them.

Our pleasures are so few and far between now and at times it's so very difficult to see a bright future. I worry all the time that things might not turn out for Robby and me, the way we dream now because of a long separation. And yet he's told me so many times that I'm the only girl he'd every marry or ever want to and he's been more faithful than any girl could expect a man to be. It's going to be difficult for both of us to adjust to a new life again. He's as restless and fidgety as I am but maybe if we can ever live a normal life again it won't be too hard. I know I'll never be content until I am married and can settle down.

We had a treat here the other day. Bing Crosby was here in person, and he visited all the wards and talked to all the boys then cracked some jokes and sang a couple numbers for us. He came at 11 o'clock in the morning so I lost some sleep, but it was worth it. He sure was swell and the GI's sure gave him a great welcome.

It's now 5 o'clock and time to get on the ball and clean this tent up before breakfast. Just finished drinking some hot chocolate which I make out of our D ration bars and condensed milk. The boys come here for their 3 o'clock break but tonight everyone was late as we've all been busy.

Here come the Penicillin boys—a couple of NCOs who go around to all the wards every 4 hours and give our wounded their Penicillin shots—that newest drug which is saving so many lives. The GI's call them the "bayonet crew" because it has to be given with a long needle.

You probably know that our war bonds are being canceled so am going to increase my Class E allotment and try to get those others straightened out because they've been taking $37.50 out of my check every month since I increased my bonds. Heck everything gets so mixed up and sometimes I don't even care—everything seems so unimportant now except saving lives, and you know that is out of our hands, too, so much of the time.

Our foot lockers are stored in Eng., and soon as this is over, they're going to try to do something about them. I sure hope we see them again cause everything I value is in mine—Robby's letters, my good watch, and my Val-Pack.

Gosh, sure don't have any luggage now except a dirty old duffle bag which is rotting because of all the dampness. We'll all look like sad sacs when we finish here but hope we can get some place to replace some worn out and mildewed clothes.

All the pts. are awake so guess I'll have to close until next time.

Your loving GI daughter,

Mary

***

Both Poncho and Redmond were three years younger than Mary, but when they walked into Medical Tent on the night of September 22, anyone would have guessed their age to be around 40. Redmond would be gone by October 1, attached to his former unit for the next big move toward Belgium. It worried Mary "no end," but out loud, for his sake, she told him that he'd be fine since all the really ugly fighting was probably all but over. Wasn't she lucky that he'd spent his convalescence learning how to be the best ward boy ever, other than Poncho, of course.

The 39th processed their 4,000th patient on September 26, 1944.[2] In a September 24 letter addressed only to her mother, Mary described their conditions and their state of mind that week in Vertus:

I'm sitting on my bunk. It's about 8 p.m. and so dark outside you can't see your hand in front of your face. It's blowing and raining and so darned cold in here we're about to have a chill. And that isn't all—trying to write a letter with a flickering candle on my left and a dim flashlight on my right is no joke. It's so breezy in here the candle just fell over and scorched my blanket. Now I suppose you're wondering why I even try to write a letter. Well, in the first place I've been neglecting you, but you'll have to blame that on this darned war—and in the second place there's nothing to do but write letters as it's too early to go to bed. In spite of a long 12 hr. day (I finally got off nites), we just can't come right off duty and go to bed. Have showers at 7:30 and it was too cold tonite, but tomorrow nite will have to go over so I can do some washing. We have to hang our washing out after dark as it gets dark at 7:30 now as the time changed again. Then we pray that it will dry in a couple of days, but it's been raining all week, and I'm down to my last pair of socks. My shoes are so heavy with mud they feel like gunboats for sure now. As you've probably guessed by now my spirits are

---

2   "39th Evacuation Hospital Unit History." WW2 US Medical Research Centre. Medical Research Center Staff Compilers, 2007. Web. March 9, 2016. https://www.med-dept.com/unit-histories/39th-evacuation-hospital/

none too high tonite, but this darned uncomfortable living is getting on everyone's nerves and yet we ought to be darned thankful we're not sweating out this horrible war in foxholes.

No wonder so many of our boys crack up. Between the horrible suffering, distorted minds, and death I've witnessed in 9 weeks it's almost more than one can take, but we can't let it get us down. And the only thing I pride myself on is that I've never revealed my inner thoughts or moods on duty. Gee, they call me their angel of Mercy. Our own boys call me the "Sweetheart of the 39th." Now all this bragging probably sounds wicked but honestly Mom, I don't mean it that way. You see it's the only compensation there is for long hours of hard work. Well, self-confidence and a wonderful feeling that I'm actually doing my part. I only wish I could tell you every one of my experiences. I'm sure my life has been as full as any girl's could be excepting of course being a wife and mother. Now that's all I want but at times it's very difficult to imagine that that dream will ever come true—when you love a man like I do and your whole future seems to be centered on that one person and then not to hear from him for almost a month, well it's as we say here—it's rough! No, I don't worry about his love or devotion for me waning or altering because by now I think I know the male sex well enough to be able to tell who's sincere and who isn't, and Robby certainly has done a wonderful job of proving his love to me. I feel sure that he's over here and fighting but my gosh, Mom, when I see these tank casualties come in so badly burnt and what not and so delirious you want to cry—well I just get sick and weak wondering if some day my sweetheart will be among them.

Mother, I wonder how many girls in this world have the beautiful memories of the most wonderful friendship and love affair which belong to me. Someday I'll tell you the story—but golly, Mom, no matter how beautiful they are you can't live on memories.

It's the sad present and uncertain future which we have to face with as much courage as we can muster and there's no use in trying to evade it or escape it. I try to do my best every day and yet so many times I feel that I've failed. And sometimes I wonder if this is really me or if I'm living in a dream. I think of you all so much and the wonderful job you and Daddy did in bringing 3 girls up. That environment that I lived in for 21 years has stood me in good stead. At least I have the reputation of being a lady here—have had some long conversations with various of our officers here who have families back home and some of them are just like big brothers and fathers to me. They call me their little girl, and no one calls me Lt. Balster anymore except the Colonel…

Well, Mom, I guess I've raved on and not said much and now the guns are booming, my candle is getting low, and I want to save part of it for tomorrow nite. My feet are so cold I can't wiggle my toes anymore so guess the best thing to do is to crawl in my sleeping bag and try to get warm…

Good nite, Mother dear, I wish I could kiss you and Daddy good nite like I used to. Will write as soon as possible again.

Your loving GI Girl,
Mary

CHAPTER 21

Toul

When he whispered to whichever favorite nurse he saw first, whether it was Alabama, Mona, or Mary, Poncho's dark irises bounced horizontally across bloodshot sclera to tell his listener the latest rumor.

When there was good news, he looked like a child who'd just discovered that he'd gotten a pony for Christmas. He announced that they'd be taking over a French hospital that had been occupied by German officers only weeks before. After having endured muddy, rain-drenched tents and a backlog of patients, finally the unit would be living in real buildings. They would be in Toul by October 1.

> … We arrived yesterday and right after dinner we set to work, and I do mean work. A civilian hospital has to be clean, but a GI hospital has to be super clean. The Colonel, Major, and Chief Nurse inspect every inch every morning. And so, every morning it's a rat race to get ready for inspection. It was bad in tents but now with floors to scrub, windowsills, cupboards, and equipment to wash every day… and every morning every doorknob, water faucet and any other brass that might be around must be polished with our special brass polish. The boys are so darned cute—they gripe like the dickens…
>
> Our living quarters consist of a house with shutters and French windows as is found in every building in France. The parlor has beautiful lavender velvet drapes, a lovely piano, real rugs, and some stuffed furniture. Our rooms are crowded—there are six in ours but after a tent it looks like paradise. Unlike the English, the French are more modern. They're living in the 20th century too while the British are still somewhere back in the 14th I believe. Anyway, they love beauty as do the English, but they believe in comfort too. Our rooms have gorgeous marble fireplaces, but what intrigues us are the radiators which actually give forth that precious stuff called heat. As far as cleanliness is concerned, the English are thorough and super clean from top to bottom, the French look lovely on top, but one doesn't have to dig very far down to find the dirt. I've been in a couple homes where the latrine adjoins the kitchen with no door in between and some actually have fowl running around inside their homes. As you know they're affectionate and demonstrative and practically worship the Americans…
>
> Captain W said he sent a couple of souvenirs to you—don't ask me why, but he's just one of those fellows who can't do enough for someone he likes. He's in Belgium now…

In her brown checkered seersucker, Alabama posed on the bed as if she were being photographed for an ad in the latest publication of *Charm*.[1] And Mona was wearing her dimples again, their return most likely the result of the prospect that the mail bag she carried may contain a letter from her new major. After a two-day hunt, Sgt. Parent had found the mail. Mona dumped their stash on Mary's bed, and the three sorted through the contents in a frenzy. Mary got seven, five of them from Robby and two from back home. Alabama had five from Mountain Brook, and Mona received two from Major Bryson, the second one stating that he'd be able to take a few hours to visit her if their newest post wasn't more than two hours from his.

Letters to St. Paul summarized news that Mary had received from Robby:

> ... Robby is in France, and I was thrilled to pieces yesterday when I received five letters from him written 1, 2, 3, 4, 5 of October and noting his new APO, thinking he must not be very far, but I don't just dare let my hopes get too high cause I sure hate disappointments. He sent me a cute picture of him and one of his buddies. It looks just like those pictures of you, Daddy, in the last war. He also sent me a bunch of candles I had asked for almost a month ago... golly, his letters are the sweetest things I've ever read. I can just almost hear him saying the words that he writes in that sweet Rebel brogue. You'll love the way he talks, and you know the Southerners' every other word is honey or baby or precious. Robby says he hasn't dated a girl since we were together and won't until he can carry his own wife out. And I believe him. He's the only man I've ever put all my faith and trust in except you, Daddy... All I know is that I'm a lucky girl to have a man like that. But when I think of the slim chance that we have of getting our happiness it scares me. If only we weren't so close and didn't know what was going on but to see the terrible casualties pour in day after day—well, you just wonder if there is any future for our generation. It's not only their wounds but what it's doing to their minds—handsome American boys scarred for life. I always think of their mothers, wives, and sweethearts back home, and that's the first thing they think of too. And these youngsters—some of them don't even shave yet—I love to take care of them best of all—they just look up to us like we could make them well. One 18 yr. old last nite who has been up front for a month now said what he wanted most was some chocolate—even a D bar so am going to bring him one tonite. We're very short on chocolate now—get one D bar a week, and it's sort of rough on sweet toothed Americans...
>
> Sat. nite finally got a nite off—the first whole nite off I've had in France... and was invited to some officers' bivouac area just behind the lines. There were 3 couples, and we went up in the command car and had fried chicken and French-fried potatoes and fresh tomatoes. There was constant firing but there we were in a pyramidal tent with an electric light, a stove, and a radio in it, enjoying supper and conversation while the battle was raging. Had special permission to be out until 11. The new rule is that everyone has to be in his own area by 8 PM now which isn't a bad idea because it's certainly not safe around these parts, and I'm such a fraidy cat I don't like to be out after blackout. If I was with Robby, I'd

---

1   *Charm* was an iconic fashion and beauty magazine in the 1940s and 1950s. At Fort Leonard Wood, Mary asked her younger sister Connie to send her a specific edition of *Charm* that featured a patient's sister. She was a model for Pond's Hand Crème, for which the caption read, "She's engaged. She's lovely. She uses Pond's."

feel safe but any other man—well, I just won't go out on a date unless we go with a group or another couple. Men will be men and are only human but men in combat—well, I feel sorry for every one of them cause it's for sure they don't know what tomorrow holds but don't ever worry that my sympathy will ever get the best of me…

Went to a German cemetery and read all the inscriptions—each grave is marked with a large black cross with a white swastika painted in the center. It has been very well kept. Most of the boys were very young. We kept walking and climbed some fences and found an exploded land mine and then came to an orchard with blue plumbs and piled our helmets with them.

It's now 3:30 AM and I'm sitting in the ward listening to the radio and gee does the music ever make me homesick. Every once in a while we hear the German propaganda and it's wicked.

Felt so rotten tonite that after midnite decided to take 40 winks. Have 2 nurses reporting to me and some extra ward boys—when we get real busy surgical and shock teams come in to help. Anyway, I laid down, but sleep was futile with patients hollering for a nurse every 2 minutes. The payoff was one wanting his face washed at 2 o'clock in the morning, another wanted to know where he could get a watch, someone else has been trying to take a hill all by himself and has been cursing the Krauts to fare thee well.

Earlier in the evening sent one of my boys down to the room where we have the PWs to spray them all with the stuff we use for lice. Then had him shave one of the boy's heads who was discovered to be full of lice today. They all have such darn long hair and when he started to shave the fellow's head, they all got excited and made an awful racket. The next thing I know the ward boy was calling for me and I tore down to see what was the matter, and they were all having a fit because they thought they were all going to have their own long hair cut off.

Most of them are scared to death—they don't know what it is to be treated kindly, I guess. They always call "Schwester" because they're afraid of our boys. Sometimes I don't know whether to hate them or what. Everything about this war is very confusing…

After the gals had been lavishing in their quarters in Toul for several days, Mona's eyes twinkled. They had cause for celebration: Major Bryson arrived. Mona hadn't gotten the opportunity to see Bryson since the night the restaurant burned down in Nogent-sur-Seine, so she was anxious to accept a date from him. And W had returned from Belgium earlier that same day. Naturally, Major Bryson didn't share specifics regarding his whereabouts, and he was to head somewhere else the next day (the gals guessed Belgium).

Mona wanted Mary and W to tag along with her and the major for the evening.

Truth be known, Mary had wanted to turn in early, but Mona had been giddy, ever since the day she got the letters from the major. Her happiness was paramount, and Mary wasn't going to spoil the moment with selfishness. She couldn't turn down a stranger, much less her best friend.

Obviously, the men were in the mood for a stupendously adventurous evening—they showed up in an open jeep in clattering rain. Even though the two officers assured the gals that the weather was clearing, they ran back inside to grab their overcoats and buckle shoes.

The men's forecast turned out to be spot-on, and soon after the clouds dissipated the moon showed up. The major and Mona cast dreamy glances toward each other. They reminded Mary of her and Robby on the *Andes* when the moon had been so fat and fecund.

What a charmed spell the moon had brought that night, but that was eight months ago. For everybody in the ETO, it might as well have been a lifetime.

> … we went jeep riding. By that time the rain had stopped and there was a moon and just as we were trying to forget the war, Bedcheck Charlies started to drone overhead, and the flak started to fly, and we got out of the jeep and went into the ditch laughing like it was funny… We sank in mud up to our knees and what I mean it was rough… It's queer but I'm just past being scared. Right now, the artillery fire is enough to disturb anyone that wasn't used to it…

October 19, 1944

> … I really intend to finish this letter today and mail it first thing in the morning. Just got off duty (I'm on "days" now) and not only do I have a pile of washing including my hair but also at least 25 letters to write but my family comes first, and you and Robby are the only ones I've written to the past two weeks. That nite duty really wore me out this time…

> Yesterday afternoon got off at 3 and went for a long walk and took some snaps. Then went over to the mess and came back here in the evening and played the piano, cards, and talked. No one had anything to drink, and I was very happy since I really hate all of it except the champagne… It hurts me to see some of these good-looking healthy Americans trying to forget war and their troubles nite after nite… some of them have reason… the boys who've been up front, get wounded and then have to face it all over again. The tales they tell make your hair stand on end, but golly just can't let it get us down. And while they're here we try to make it as pleasant as possible for them. I have the cutest little 19 yr. old patient. He was up front for 71 days until finally he got a serious case of gout. He hasn't had a haircut for so long I told him I was going to bring my curlers over and fix him up. His attitude is marvelous, but he's such a baby. I don't mean he ever complains. He's just sweet. He's from Ky. and when I asked him if he wore shoes 'fore he came into the army he said no and he had to put pebbles in his GI shoes when he came in just to feel at home. These youngsters can always get you one better every time. They're taking it much better than the older men, some of whom get very despondent and it's hard to pull them out of it. I guess we are morale builders all right because they respond beautifully to a smile or just a little favor. Today I bathed a chaplain who has a partial body cast and tried to do my best for him. And when he said, "Mary I feel so good now and thank you very much," well, what more can a nurse ask for. Monetary reward doesn't count as far as I'm concerned any more—it's the wonderful feeling that we've made someone's life a bit happier thru our efforts. Thanks, Mom and Dad, for everything you've ever done for me but mostly for helping me stick to the career that was always my dream and without your financial as well as the other encouraging help you gave me, I could not have had my dream come true.

> Now if you will just keep praying for Robby and me and the future that we want so badly I just won't ever ask another thing. I guess I want too much out of life, but I've found one doesn't get anything unless it's pursued, and I intend to pursue my other dream of Robby and a family as I did the career one, and I guess if God wills it, it will be fulfilled someday also.

I guess you wonder how I can ramble on the way I do, but you know one doesn't get a chance to speak one's inner thoughts here and besides thoughts like the above should only be spoken to those you love and who know you better than you do yourself...

October 28, 1944

... Got a beautiful letter from that wonderful man of mine last nite, and he said he sent you some perfume, Mom, so you sure should stink pretty when it catches up with you. Have you ever received the other from Captain W? Golly, he keeps writing to me, and I wish he would forget about me, but I hate to hurt anyone's feelings, so I just answer his letters every now and then...

October 31, 1944

Dearest Daddy,

Upon receiving your letter of the 15th sort of gathered you'd like a letter just for you, so I will try to bring you up to date on latest events here. Personally, as far as the war is concerned believe you know as much if not more as to how things are going than we do, although there are radios, bulletin boards and plenty of 1st hand information from boys just back from the front. But we just hardly discuss the war around here. Every evening when we entertain our officer friends the main topic of conversation is the home front, the life we left behind and how very wonderful it will be to be a civilian again. The consensus at present is that politics are holding up things here, the general feeling is also a bitter one because why should those war lovers sit back in our U.S. and just let this mess go on while boys are dying and sweating it out in their cold muddy foxholes existing on cold K rations and wondering why they have to be there. We're all so very tired of it and want to come home so badly, but there's just not a darned thing any of us can do but wait and wait for orders and then carry them out to the best of our ability. Perhaps none of this makes sense to you and I certainly have no right to try to talk about it, so I'll just quit now and get down to something else which is at least more pleasant to read.

We are still in our comfortable quarters and can't even guess what the next move will be. Today started another training program—my aching back, now we all detest them—drills, calisthenics, classes, but they have to keep us occupied I guess, until things start popping again.

Gosh, Dad, I don't guess France is any cleaner than it was the last war. In fact, I don't see how the people can stay healthy and live in such filth. Am referring mostly to the sanitation system if there is one. Thank goodness our army is on the ball and gives us our typhoid shots and purifies our drinking water or we would all be sick or dead. The water that comes from these faucets contains little lumps of dirty matter and it smells awful. We felt a thousand times cleaner in the field because then every bit of water for drinking and washing was G.I. water. This stuff is swimming with typhoid, and we're not even allowed to brush our teeth with it.

... Time out to fix the blackouts. Here we have shutters and rubber sheets to make our blackout effective. I often wonder what it will be like to walk down a lighted street again.

The boys are cleaning their guns as they do every evening about this time and this whole house just shook.

The weather the past weeks reminds me so much of home. There's frost now and the trees are beautiful and there's a harvest moon, but here we call it a bomber's moon... Robby fussed at me for not writing very cheerful letters home in a very nice way and I know he's right, so I'll try to do better. He warned me of telling everything I've seen and heard and he's right there too. Anyway, if you think this letter includes anything that may worry Mom just keep it from her.

There is really no sense in worrying about me, tho, because I'm around many friends and believe it or not can almost take care of myself now.

… Just happened to think in 3 more months we will have earned two gold stripes to wear on our sleeves. Have already earned 3 stars for our E and O ribbon for various places of combat where we've been. I don't care if we don't earn any more stripes or stars or anything else. Just so we can come home soon is all we ask.

Good nite, Daddy, and here's a great big kiss from your soldier.

Lovingly,

Mary

November 1, 1944

Dearest Mom,

This is going to be a request letter so please be prepared. Have been sitting here in the dining room drinking tea and gossiping with some of the girls and the conversation got around to Xmas gifts. As I've been racking my brain for something for Robby finally got an idea. It's a man's identification bracelet. Please try to have one made with the following inscription…

And now for some personal requests. Would you please write to Lord and Taylor—New York and ask them to send you COD 3 light tan—rayon-silk shirts which they carry for army nurses. That is, they did when were there in Feb. I bought one and it's about worn out from washing and ironing. Have them send 2 size 34 and 1 size 36. Then when you receive them if you will wrap each one separately and send them 1st class air mail, they will arrive much faster. Also, would you try to get Mona and me each an OD tie? They look super with the light shirts.

Now this next one perhaps you won't be able to fulfill, but if you can please do. I don't know whether you still have to have coupons for shoes and if you do, skip it, but I would like very much a comfortable pair of oxfords. The ones I got in St. Louis are worn out and these GI shoes are about to kill my feet. The ones I got in St. Louis were Enna Jetticks—size 8A, British tan and I really don't care what make they are, just so they're comfortable. After wearing field shoes for so long my feet are wider than they used to be, but I don't seem to need much length.

Also, if you could find some nice hosiery would appreciate it—size 10. And as usual Kleenex, food, and any other bright ideas you have.

Send me the bill and I will reply with a money order immediately.

Expect to leave here in very short order and won't mind cause male complications are getting too much for me. Don't misunderstand—there's only one man as far as I'm concerned but they've been ganging up on me lately. Last nite stood a fellow up and he and his crowd got angry with me, but he and his friends came over anyway with some chickens which we fried, and Capt. W made some super cole slaw with olives in it, and Mona's friend brought champagne and we had white bread and fresh butter. There are 12 of us in my regular crowd—6 officers and 6 girls and we've really had some nice times—mostly playing cards, dancing, and eating.

Am stiff as a board today from calisthenics so you see guess I needed some. Must close and get ready for chow—more later.

Your loving GI girl

Mary

CHAPTER 22

These Boys

By the second week of November, chronic depression transfixed each member of the unit. Thoughts of having no future with anyone had been lingering in their subconscious minds and disrupting sleep. They began to identify and live with the fear their patients had been living with for months. The possibility of no future had turned into a reality—it used to be a fleeting thought that could be put away like a bad penny. But by mid-November, it was always there.

Mary's mental struggles centered around an obsessive worrying about Robby that was most likely connected to guilt. When the two shared those 10 days on the *Andes*, there'd been an excessive need to belong to someone. It was natural. They were going to war. Who knew what their future would bring? In her mind, only God knew. She had a psychological need to find answers during a confusing and unsure time. If she could belong to someone as safe as this "shave tail," who was the all-American ideal of bravery, patriotism, and a boastful hope that the Allies would win the war, well then, what else could a gal ask for in life? To commit to Robby was to commit to a future. To be physically attracted to him was just a bonus.

And when it came to ideals and morally sound values, Robby was the southern version of her father, a true gem among so many men who'd disappointed her, like Clinton, who apparently found another gal in Boca, and even Zim, whose letters had begun dwindling in number soon after the 39th had been sent on Tennessee maneuvers. But Robby's devotion to her had never waned. His love had been steady, dependable, and it didn't seem to matter how many months the war separated them; when he was able, he wrote to her every day. When Sgt. Parent came back from a mail-finding mission, everyone who knew Mary teased her that the sergeant had labeled one bag "Lt. Balster," because there were so many letters from her beau Robby. Robby meant a larger connection for her. He belonged to the army. He understood service like her father. He had an incredibly infectious personality, and he offered hope for two reasons. He was one of those "glass half-full" types, *and* he was not a part of the 39th. Not knowing his situation or station or experiences in the war helped Mary's outlook. He could remain idolized and idealized. She could worship him because he was the paragon of American strength, patriotism, and grit. She made him her ideal, and though the actual number of days they'd spent together had been few, he never ventured from the mold she'd cast him in. Guilt forced her to obsess about his safety, for underneath the longing she had for spending the rest of her life with this ideal, she believed that fate would punish her. Fantasies of spending a future with Robby wouldn't be allowed to become real because of her continual romantic feelings for W.

But by the second week of November, she hadn't received a letter from Robby since those five that had arrived in Toul. Many of her friends had continued to hear from their beaus who also served in First Army. Of course, First Army was massive, and Paul Ferreria, the logistics expert for the 39th who'd been one of Robby's pals and had bunked with him in their stateroom on the *Andes*, reminded her that Robby may not even be in First Army anymore, that even in late August Robby had suspected that there would be a change in his attachment.

In the meantime, Mary's ability to contain her attraction for W was waning. He'd insisted that she go with him to see Marlene Dietrich entertain over at TUSA Headquarters. It was an extraordinary day, as it made Mary feel special to be the only nurse from the 39th in the presence of such glamour and grace. And it seemed that W carried as much style as Marlene. He was like a doctor version of Cary Grant.

At the same time, her capacity for envisioning any future with Robby was rapidly disappearing, and she was far past seeing W as an emotional crutch. By November she would become disappointed, almost despondent, if W received orders to teach surgical techniques to clinical personnel at other evacs. And each time he was away, he never failed to write her.

As emotionally wrecked as Mary felt, she told herself that she was faring better than Mona. Since Major Bryson had left for Belgium, Mona's luster faded. She couldn't even find the energy or the wherewithal to force her voice above a whisper. Her gait was as slow as an old woman's. Mary thought it a very bad sign when she realized that Mona had become so depressed that she now seemed addicted to it. She held onto it like Silas Marner held on to his coins, for goodness' sakes; her emotional state had deteriorated into some sort of obsessive need to hoard despair. She held onto mental suffering like a cursed treasure. It was so unhealthy.

To get her mind off worrying over Mona, she decided to write her father.

November 14, 1944
Dearest Daddy,

It's 4 a.m. and as most of the boys are sleeping, guess I can take some time out for a couple of letters if I don't fall asleep myself...

Last night between 7 and 10 we admitted eighty patients to our ward. I'm glad their mothers and their loved ones can't see their boys as they come to us. They're cold, hungry, muddy from head to foot, their clothes are torn and they're sick to death of foxholes with inadequate clothing and shoes. Our enemy has outsmarted us when it comes to protecting their soldiers' feet—they have big rubber boots—our boys have GI shoes which aren't much protection especially when they can't take their shoes off for days at a time, and then when they finally do get a chance many of them have developed "Trench Foot," disabling most of them for combat and for life.

Maybe if it continues to be cold and wet and our boys will continue to get not only battle wounds and Trench Foot and pneumonia and the number of combat exhaustion cases increases, and a few thousand more people back home receive messages from the War Dept., like "Missing in Action," etc., and maybe if the government decides they can't afford to give any more purple hearts and oak leaf clusters and silver stars—maybe then someone will put a stop to this cruel and senseless war.

And something else while I'm on the subject—you know, Daddy, if our boys don't get their jobs back and have all the things they've been told they're fighting for, the people in the U.S. are going to see what war is like because these boys are not the boys that left home, although because they're Americans I guess, they can still laugh and joke and tease and hand out that famous Yankee line which really never gets tiresome, although I hear it every day of my life. But there's something else that you don't discover until you listen to these soldiers and learn that there is bitterness and hatred in their minds, too, because they've seen their best buddy killed and because the best years of their lives are being spent in a useless way. It's going to take time to heal those mental scars, and I guess there will probably be enough of those that may prevent another war for a few years anyway...

I hear the familiar sound of a Jerry plane above us, but when it's right overhead we don't worry much about it—it's those that may be following him that we can't hear that are the cause for concern, but what we don't know doesn't hurt us. We all realize, though, that the Luftwaffe is not washed up yet...

It's been six weeks since I've heard from Robby, and I don't know what to think. There was some talk about him getting transferred to a less dangerous job. Golly, I hope that happened and the transfer is why I haven't heard anything. Better I should change the subject before I start crying.

By the third week of November, perpetual rains harnessed General Patton's blustery offensive. But it did offer the 39th the opportunity to catch up to some of his troops. They traveled piecemeal to the Heinrich Himmler Barracks in Morhange, just east of Toul, and were ready to receive the latest band of sick and wounded by November 22.

On Thanksgiving Day, November 23, at 0200, German 280mm shells hit and shook the Heinrich Himmler barracks. The supply room and laundry were destroyed from the blasts, and, as if they did not have enough to do, the 39th admitted 98 patients due to the shelling. Everyone assured each other that the German barrage was "just a fluke," surely not a harbinger.

That November day became an emotional dividing line for the 39th. Every day past November 23, 1944, held a distinctly heavy memory of exhaustion so extreme that no one seemed to be able to find any emotions. Mona and Mary discovered this phenomenon during a conversation they shared at the Thanksgiving meal. It seemed so strange. They began to laugh at the fact that they longed for those first days in France back in the summer when they were so scared. They had been talking about the feeling of "emptiness" that they both were experiencing at the present and began to look around the mess tent. Everyone else who was eating turkey in that tent also looked… what, they wondered. They looked, for lack of a better description—*incomplete*. Everybody's faces seemed to be washed in a white pallor with deep-socketed eyes, dry and half-closed. Their shoulders slumped over their food with little interest in eating, although they forced smiles to show their deep appreciation for all who were attempting to give them a decent Thanksgiving feast. But something was missing.

Then Mary and Mona decided what it was. Everybody was searching for fear because fear was something to feel. They wanted to own that tangible feeling of fear. Anything was better than the malaise they felt (and wore) at present.

The only physical feeling they had left was shivering, the result of a bitterly cold rain that descended on Morhange. Three weeks later, the rain left, and heavy snow took its place. Patton asked every chaplain in Third Army to begin praying for more favorable weather.

CHAPTER 23

Snow Globe

During the early afternoon of December 10, 1944, Mary looked about the Heinrich Himmler barracks on her walk toward the mess tent. It seemed as if all inanimate objects belonging to the 39th were now draped in a white velour blanket. When she entered to grab any snacks that the boys might enjoy for their usual 3:00 a.m. break, she stood over the long table, contemplating whether she should snack on fruitcake or popcorn. The Red Cross had been on the beam with treats lately.

Poncho bounced in with new hope and a wide smile. There was a guy who looked a lot like Mary's picture of Robby who just drove up in a jeep with a chaplain. But it couldn't really be him, Poncho said, because Robby's doppelganger looked to be a first lieutenant—unless, of course, maybe Mary forgot to mention that Robby had been promoted?

Mary was exhausted. She was in no mood to be teased.

Then Poncho asked her if she had her lipstick in her pocket.

Of course, but why was Poncho barking on so?

He took her by the elbow and led her outside.

There they were, Robby and a chaplain, climbing up a few snowy steps that led to Major Scanlon's office.

"Robby!" she cried.

He placed his hand on his chaplain friend's shoulder to gesture that he should go on ahead.

He stepped back down into the plush carpet of snow and opened his arms for Mary to dive into him. With chapped, ruddy cheeks, she tromped through the mounds resembling a tiny figure trapped in a snow globe. Her will to reach him overcame the fragility of her frame. In seconds, she regained all the moxie that war had taken from her. She threw herself into Robby with such force that both lost their balance. They plunged into a snow mound locked in an embrace. Robby's composure and typical GI sensibilities abandoned him. They frolicked and giggled and tumbled about in the snow mounds kissing and hugging and kissing again.

Robby lifted himself up from the snow and extended his hand to help Mary to her feet. Then he cupped his gloved hands around her diminutive face.

"Let me get a good look at 'cha," he teased.

She'd dropped 15 pounds. And six months of war and a bout of malaria had been responsible for Robby's 20-pound loss.

In the black stuff of space, clouds draped the moonlight for the mere three hours that Robby was there. But just as he and his buddy made their way to the jeep, lumps of clouds dissolved like sugar in hot water. Stars and a full moon lit the night and increased the likelihood of night bombers raiding and strafing, leaving Robby's fate to the will of multiple forces, none of which he could control. Later she said, "Well, there was nothing to do. It was war."

> December 11, 1944
> Dearest Family,
>
> Have big news for you tonite—last evening… who should be waiting for me but Robby. Golly, I practically went into shock and still haven't recovered. He was here for just 3 hours as he had driven quite a ways and had to get back last nite, and besides I had to be on duty although one of my pals relieved me until 9. He had a friend with him, so we didn't get to talk over so many things that I had wanted to… As usual after he left, I broke down as I always have when we're together and this time it was worse since he is going into combat… So far, he is just the same, but no one can deny that I haven't changed along with the rest of… the outfit. It just can't be helped—seeing young boys suffer day after day… I'm so head over heels in love with Robby, and he has to go into battle, and then I have the terrible feeling of guilt that's just sort of torturing me. Robby hasn't dated a single girl since we were together in England in June… I try to rationalize and say I couldn't stand to sit in every nite and that it helps to be able to forget the trials of the day for a few hours. But if Robby can do it, to be worthy of his love and devotion, know I should too.

During a period of less than 24 hours, she'd gone from not feeling any emotions at all to feeling elation and pure joy when she shared those hours with Robby, and then on to extreme anxiety about their future. Then it occurred to her that when her personal life took a turn, regardless if that turn was enviable or not, she always could count on a larger force pressing her to think beyond her own joys or sufferings. Maybe it was God's way of tapping her on the shoulder to remind her of the real reason she was on the earth—to serve those in dire need of her skills.

Whatever the force was, it came to call. On December 12, the 39th admitted 119 patients, then 151 the next day. On December 14 admissions seemed light by comparison with 104. On December 15, there were 122 more.[1] The statistics would not wane. On December 16, the Germans were going for broke in the Ardennes.

---

1   "39th Evacuation Hospital Unit History." WW2 US Medical Research Centre. Medical Research Center Staff Compilers, 2007. Web. March 9, 2016. https://www.med-dept.com/unit-histories/39th-evacuation-hospital/

CHAPTER 24

Redmond

During those miserable days the 39th could not move. There was no break in the weather. Blood plasma supplies were dwindling. Mary, Mona, and Alabama and certainly every nurse, medic and physician prayed for a miracle. Being understaffed had never bothered them, but to be undersupplied seemed unconscionable. Last summer speculation had centered around the possibility of medical supplies running low if the war couldn't find an end by winter. Now their worst fears were not only their new reality but were much worse than what they'd imagined.

Mary had little time for sleep or correspondence, but at 5:00 a.m. she managed to finish a letter that she'd begun writing to her parents the night before, dated December 18, 1944:

… Just came back from taking a shower and now am sitting by the oil stove drying my hair before I go to chow. Mona is still in bed, so I just got a pail of water, and I'm heating it for her. She hardly ever gets up in time to take a shower that's from 4–5 for nite nurses but boy I wouldn't miss it. Got up at 2 today and washed clothes and ironed my fatigues. They finally got the generator working so we have lights now—blinking lights I should say as they keep going off and on and it takes forever to iron anything.

Last night the rush started at 9 p.m. and we never sat down once after that except for chow. The wounds were terrible, and the poor boys scared and wet and cold. We were busy giving hypos and repairing dressings etc. and as we are the admitting ward the backlog is terrific. One little 19-year-old boy received a back wound so had to lie on his stomach and when I went to give him a hypo his nose was just dripping, and he couldn't use his hands because they were wrapped in gauze and strapped along his sides, so I got some dressings to use for hankies and just had him blow his nose until it was all clean. Remember how you used to say, "now, blow," Mom? Well, I felt just like a mother then. He said, "gee nurse, thanks a lot," and the tears were rolling down his cheeks.

I hate myself for griping about my own little troubles and feel so ashamed when I see our boys come in like that nite after nite.

Well, like the Capt. said last nite it is up to our generation to make the supreme sacrifice and we can only hope that it will be a sacrifice that will be great enough so that our children won't have to do it 20 years from now, if there *is* enough of our generation left to *have* children. I mean the kind that will make good American citizens because we all know that the cream of the crop is being destroyed in this war. I know I'm no better or don't deserve to have my man spared in this war any more than the millions of others who have lost theirs, but I pray every day that Robby will come out of this whole in body and mind, and maybe God will let us have our happiness someday.

Mary noticed that Mona still wasn't up. She'd committed to a habit of wrapping herself up in that damn stinking sleeping bag until five minutes before she had to report to duty. And she was hardly eating.

Mary had to do something. How could she help her? If only she could get her to talk about it. But Mona wasn't ever much of a talker about her own problems.

"Mona, are you awake? I need to tell you something," Mary said, weakly. She was.

"Look, I have an idea. I'm going to run to chow. Get a huge breakfast for us to share. I won't be long. Someone said they found some hot chocolate powder in a crate. I'll bring some back. I've got the fire going really well. Watch it for me, would you?"

"Sure, Mary."

"Oh, look, Mona, one more thing. Have you been able to keep up with your service diary any? I just wondered. Since you're awake, here it is. You can use the beautiful pen that Robby brought me when he was here. It writes so smoothly. Try it out. I'll be back soon, okay?"

Mona stirred and opened her eyes fully.

Mary would be expecting to see her with pen in hand when she returned.

She took the pen and muttered, "Oh, hell, okay. God damn it." Mary was so sweet. She'd force herself to indulge her.

There's one way to win war in the middle of the 20th century—through attrition of human capital, expendable human flesh, and the only difference in who wins is if you, as commanding officer, can expend a little less flesh than your enemy. For generals, sending 18-year-olds to charge a hill that rains bullets from machine guns to dip and dive into the dirt or through their bodies isn't only the expectation, it's the goal. Age is irrelevant. Station, also irrelevant.

But you, 18-year-old, you volunteered, so you believe that you should survive because, out of some sort of bizarre sense of entitlement, wouldn't the gods show you favor over the chap beside you who didn't volunteer? The one who was conscripted because he wasn't as patriotic or as responsible? The problem with that thought is that you no longer own an individuality, a personal history, a life worth saving so that you can go home one day and raise a family in a peaceful world. You are part of a war machine, and no matter your age or station, you are expendable.

You are not in the least important to anyone other than your contribution to the collective war machine. "Fly through Normandy like shit through a goose," our famous general says. Normandy is the goose, and you are the shit.

By writing the words, Mona hoped for a catharsis. There was some relief, but the thorough cleansing she needed didn't seem to be there. She wondered for a few minutes why the words she'd written hadn't helped her all that much. Then it occurred to her.

Fear was getting in the way. She hadn't felt fear in so long she didn't recognize it at first.

If living near the front lines had taught her one thing it was to never own the audacity to expect to live another day. So, what if she was the next to die and someone found her service diary among her things? Dear God if they looked inside and saw what she'd just written, surely, they'd burn it. Or what if they mailed it to censors first, and they'd mark out these words with that penetrating black ink. Or what if the little book somehow escaped anyone's attention and was hurriedly packed and sent home? Her mother wouldn't understand. She'd think, "Oh God, what happened to my Monica? She left home so brave and loyal. How could she have turned to these thoughts—almost traitorous. What happened to my girl?"

Either way, if fate were to find favor with placing her under the next barrage, like the one that destroyed the supply room and killed the sentry, these words, left under her cot to be found later, would damage her reputation that she'd spent years molding. Dying young was easy compared to the thought of her mother misunderstanding the words she just wrote.

She ripped them from the diary and tossed them into the faint burn of dying coal that Mary's fire had become. They barely lit. She got down on her knees to stoke the papers around until a little flame caught and trapped them. Like a nurse over a restless, dying soldier, she watched over them until she was sure that they were ashes.

Now she felt a little better. She crawled back to her cot, wrapped her body into a fetal position, and found sleep that had eluded her for weeks.

***

Neither Mona nor Mary would have the time nor the inclination to write anything for 10 days. Redmond returned to the unit on December 20, the same night that Mary limped into the Surgical Ward tent to work the night shift. A "flu bug," as she had identified it, had been "raging" in her head for the past two days. Mona was there already. There was a third nurse—Laura—who was part of a surgical team that had been attached to the 39th a few months before. It was meant to be a temporary attachment, but the casualties' staggering numbers had demanded that Laura's unit remain for the unforeseen future.

Mona asked Laura to manage admissions for a few minutes while she took a look at Mary's foot. The red swelling that had never been explained those months before had returned. Mary threatened Mona with her life if she mentioned the edema to Chiefee. She'd be okay. She'd be just fine and reminded Mona that when the edema showed up it never hurt. It just made it difficult to walk as fast as she normally did. Besides, it was her head that was absolutely pounding, but that was just congestion and certainly wasn't debilitating enough to be reported. The boys were far worse off. Mona just needed to help her get the shoe back on. That was all.

Mona promised that she wouldn't say anything to Chief Maxson. They needed Mary too badly anyway. As much as it grieved her to do so, she was compelled to tell Mary about Redmond.

He'd been admitted with 40 percent of his body suffering from tank burns and had a gunshot wound to the chest. The German captain was probably removing the bullet as they spoke, but he'd need plasma, and Mona wasn't sure if there was any left.

There was no way there wasn't plasma, Mary said. She was sure of it. God wouldn't dare have pulled Redmond through the pneumonia that almost took his life last summer to put him in a Sherman five months later and him die from not enough plasma. That wasn't acceptable. There had to be some left in Supply.

Mona called out for Laura to run to what was left of the Supply room. She knew the odds of her locating any would be low. No supplies had been replenished since Supply and Laundry had been bombed on Thanksgiving Day.

Laura came back empty-handed. Mary stopped her and asked if she'd looked thoroughly. She said she had. There wasn't anything they could use. But Mary couldn't let it go. She refused to hear it and told Mona that she and Laura would be right back.

She leaned on Laura's arm to get to Supply. The damn foot was not cooperating.

"There," she remarked, then pointed to some bottles with her flashlight. Had Laura checked that crate? It looked undamaged.

She said yes, it was intact, but she'd checked the bottles in it already. They weren't the right ones. Then she said the unthinkable, the illogical, the most absurd words that Mary ever heard. The bottles were marked "colored," so they would be of no use. It was against regulation to give a white patient any plasma from a bottle that was labeled "colored."

Mary's skin seared. She made her way to the crate and leaned over it, directing the light to see the labels for herself. They did read "colored." She ripped the labels off four of the bottles and shoved them into Laura's arms, told her to run back to the ward. She'd take full responsibility for the decision, and they could court martial her for all she cared.

She screamed at her, "Boys are just boys. They're not a color, for God's sake you miserable, mindless, pathetic excuse for a…" but Laura was gone.

Mary didn't know how much Laura heard. She didn't care. And if the moron reported her for going against army regulations, so be it. But if she didn't get that plasma to Redmond's surgeon in less than two minutes, she was dead anyway. Mary would kill her.

Left alone, she bent back over the crate and tore off every label that displayed the word "colored." Her back leaned against the side of the only wall of the supply room that was still standing, then slid against it until she reached the floor.

Her mind floated into a daze. She became part of the debris that surrounded her, the glass shards, the bullet casings, the splintered wooden crates, all the used-up and shattered muck.

***

It was dusk all day long. That's all she could remember.

Mary wasn't making any sense, but that was okay. Alabama was so relieved to find her in the rubble of what used to be the Supply Room. It didn't matter what she'd just said. They'd figure that out later. Mary didn't have to worry. They'd be whippin' her right back into shape. Mary wouldn't have to do a thing but just grab on to her arm and get up and out of the mess. She promised Mary that if she could just get up, she could lean on her and limp along back to Surgical to check on that sweet boy Redmond.

"He made it?" Mary whispered, afraid to ask it out loud.

So far. But they'd have to see what the next days would bring. But right after they checked on him, they'd need to get Mary to bed before she ended up with pneumonia—if she didn't have it already.

***

As commanding officer of the 39th, Col. Bracher's main objective was to keep the unit as close to the battles as possible. It was a most frustrating job. He understood General Patton's ire over the fact that the 39th and other Third

Army evacs could not locate suitable sites fast enough to support the troops. He was angry, too. Few buildings remained in France, Belgium, Luxembourg, and Germany. The ones that could potentially become adequate to house the wounded often were in areas still too dangerous for the 39th to inhabit. When Major Scanlon and Paul Ferreria scouted areas closer to the fighting and would become hopeful that they had found a place that might work, SHAEF had often promised the site to another unit.

Just before Christmas Day, the 39th finally received permission to get closer to the troops. By December 24, the evac moved to a Catholic girls' school—St. Joseph's College in Virton, Belgium.

North of the 39th, in Bastogne, the 101st Airborne and other Allied troops were surrounded by the enemy. For a week or more they were holed up, but on December 27, General Patton's Fourth Division penetrated a mere 300-yard swath and liberated the 101st Airborne and other troops, the heroic division pushing through reputedly insurmountable winter weather under the leadership of a general who personified sheer American will. He simply refused to retreat.

Consequently, staggering numbers of casualties rocked the 39th. The unit received multiple tank burn victims like Redmond, as well as patients with bullet wounds, frost bite, and trench foot. Some had contracted pneumonia while they were surrounded. And Mary knew that the survivors would be hard-pressed to ever get out of their minds the images of their fallen brothers entombed in the death snows.

But the unit's medical personnel believed that, had it not been for General Patton, their jobs would have been relegated almost solely to counting corpses. Poncho was heard saying he believed that General Patton was the only Allied general who had the guts and fortitude to inspire the men of the Fourth Division in their liberation of Bastogne.

CHAPTER 25

General Patton's Vagabonds

Dearest Mom and Dad,
　... I just finished sweeping and mopping these cracked wooden floorboards and began building a fire. As usual I was in a hurry to get a fire started so dumped some wood and coal on. After I'd used up all my paper and kindling with no results decided maybe the stove was clogged up so emptied four trays of ashes out of the thing and dug around with my hands to get the clinkers out. By that time, I had to sweep and mop all over again but now have a beautiful fire going. Had almost decided to give up, too, but I got so mad at it that I felt just like I was fighting Germans and was determined to get the best of it, and I did, just like our boys who are going to whip those darn Krauts if it takes every man we have to do it.
　I wish that every American back home was fully aware of what we're up against and the terrible barbarous things the enemy has been doing. I guess Americans would give every penny they could spare so we could have the blood, the tires, the ammunition, etc., that's going to mean our victory and their total destruction.
　And I fully believe it will have to be total destruction if the world expects to be run democratically. You can't imagine what it would mean to have to live under our enemy's form of government until you come in contact with those who have. Better I should change the subject. Perhaps I've said too much already, but the censor may take care of it...

By the time General Patton's men had cleared Bastogne of the enemy, the 39th Evacuation Hospital had processed its 10,000th patient.[1]

On January 4, 1945, Mary received an unexpected surprise when Poncho caught up with her on the way to chow. Chief Maxson was looking for her. She asked Poncho if she was in trouble again. He said he didn't think so but that she needed to go see Lt. Maxson that day, as the Chief was planning to be gone for the next few days and wanted to see Mary before she left.

Mary decided to skip chow and head over to "face the music" from Chiefee. Her mind tried to comb through the last several days. She'd been so busy

---

1　"39th Evacuation Hospital Unit History." WW2 US Medical Research Centre. Medical Research Center Staff Compilers, 2007. Web. March 9, 2016. https://www.med-dept.com/unit-histories/39th-evacuation-hospital/

she didn't have a clue what she might have done this time. And whether Redmond could overcome the uphill battle he faced from those horrific injuries had been so difficult for her to manage emotionally. On the one hand, she was thankful for every day he got through that she didn't care if she was in trouble with Chiefee again. On the other hand, it sure would be hard to take another admonishment from Chiefee when she'd been so devoted to saving as many boys as she could, despite that darn flu bug that she was just now getting over. She just couldn't think of what she could have done to upset Chief Maxson again.

But Chiefee seemed different. Her demeanor toward Mary was "almost kind" during this brief meeting. She asked Mary to take a seat. A report had landed on her desk, a complaint of nurse incompetence. Mary was confused. Chief Maxson explained that an incompetence complaint alleged that a lack of knowledge or skill had been committed by an RN. In this case, the person who wrote the complaint said that Lt. Balster showed a lack of knowledge by ordering the writer of the complaint to take colored plasma to the surgical ward and hand it to a surgeon to be administered on white patients.

"Oh, yes. I remember now, Chief Maxson. Yes ma'am, I did that. I was beside myself. Lt. Ames had told me a few minutes before that Private Redmond had been admitted. I did get very angry."

Chief Maxson asked Mary if she had, indeed, ripped the colored labels off plasma bottles. Mary answered in the affirmative. And she added that she would do it again if any patient, "white, colored, or purple" needed the plasma. "After all, Chief Maxson, if the war has taught us anything, hasn't it taught us that boys are just boys?"

To Mary's great surprise, Chief Maxson wholeheartedly agreed. Indeed, Chief Maxson "made a big deal out of it," and ripped the complaint in two and tossed it in the garbage can.

She added that Mary's decision to defy an army-issued directive was not at all incompetent. It was heroic and that Mary's decision saved Redmond's life that night and also saved several other boys' lives. Maxson thanked Mary for making the right clinical decision, and she promised Mary that she'd write a letter of commendation when she returned from her trip to TUSA later in the week.

On January 5, Poncho arranged for Captain Maxson to ride to TUSA Headquarters via ambulance, but on the way, it slid on a patch of ice. The wreck caused her to suffer a debilitating back injury. A few days later, Poncho told Mary that Chief Maxson was going to be sent stateside for surgery. Her days in the 39th were over.

Without a chief, Dagny Solberg continued to show superior leadership skills, effectively triaging hundreds of patients through the wards of the 39th. On January 9, the unit admitted 137 patients, and for the next 10 days patient admissions continued to reach exhausting numbers.

Beginning on January 18, there was a reprieve, for two reasons. General Patton's Third Army had succeeded in pushing back the Germans close to the positions they'd held prior to December 16. Secondly, because the enemy was clearly now on the run, the Allies needed to keep up the pressure to chase the Germans back to the Rhineland, so troops were moving rapidly. All evacuation units were expected to keep the pace, but the 39th found itself far behind the troop movement and, as a consequence, patient load decreased until a recon team could scope out potential areas to move closer to the troops. They would look southeast of Brussels.

St. Hubert, Belgium, was reported to have a run-down school building that might serve to house the 39th with engineers' help. With most buildings of any size demolished, one that was only partly bombed out was now considered ideal.

The patient load was so light that Mona and Mary retreated to the Red Cross tent to scavenge snacks. They really weren't all that hungry; it was simply their way of achieving some sense of normalcy.

Snow drifts piled about like heaps of whipped cream, the result of a massive winter storm that had pounded the area just two days before. During late morning of the same day, Mona's now serious beau, Major Bryson, had been awarded a two-day leave and drove a heated jeep to the 39th.

When Mary and Mona first caught sight of him, Mary asked him if Third Army had run out of barbers for the officers, too. He threw her a half smile, embraced Mona, and said that notwithstanding the time it would take for their friend Alabama to give him a haircut, he planned to spend every minute with Mona. His appearance had shocked the gals. He'd left with a black crew cut and a thick waist. He returned from Belgium with long grey streaks of hair that looked like an old mare's matted mane. His forehead was marked with bold creases.

Later Bryson asked W about Mona's and Mary's mental states.

They were most likely suffering from mental exhaustion, but he'd only returned from Belgium earlier that day. He did know that Mona had been working double shifts until very recently. And he'd found out that Mary had ended up sick again with that strange transient edema that always seemed to plague her when she got run down or had a cold. And she'd been to the dentist over at Comm Z (Communications Zone) several times. Her teeth were falling apart because of lack of nutrition. Nevertheless, she had gotten some of her sass back. She'd been through a very tough emotional hurdle, almost losing a patient from tank burns that she'd cared for last summer, but he'd turned the corner and had been sent stateside once the unit had been able to evacuate patients a few days ago. Clearly, both gals needed a change in scenery. It would be good for both of them.

W had been thinking about taking a drive to see St. Hubert, checking the engineers' progress on make-shifting the school there. He was planning to take Mary. Without Captain Maxson lurking about, it wouldn't be a problem to free Mary and Mona out of the Virton confines for a couple of hours. Maybe Bryson and Mona wanted to tag along.

Bryson took out a map from his jeep and plotted a route, speculating that it wouldn't take the four more than an hour, an hour and a half, tops, to reach the school building.

He drove, Mona beside him; Mary and W took the back seat. The clouds had looked ominously snow-filled earlier that morning, but by the time they left the post around noon the sunrays peeked out and seemed intent on burning off the clouds. Still, Mary felt "bone cold," and she brought along four blankets, wrapping two around Mona and keeping the other two for herself. W opened the blankets for Mary to crawl in and then pulled her body to him, using his right arm to hold the blankets taut round her shoulders.

Mary's eyes darted a stern gaze at W. She didn't want any loving gestures toward her in front of Mona. She could easily turn around to say something mundane to Mary and notice the apparent emotional intimacy. Mary had continued to deny to herself, her friends, and her family her feelings for him, maintaining the stance that she considered W to be nothing more to her than a marvelously supportive surrogate older brother.

Since having been with Robby for those few hours on December 10, it had become easier to repeat the mantra to W that she fully intended to marry Robby. Of course, it helped that the patient load had kept them so busy. And with Redmond's near demise, Mary's thoughts had been consumed with his clinical needs, leaving little time to ponder her attraction to W or her devotion to Robby.

As they drove away from the 39th's present location, there was a sense that all of them had been living in a sort of psychological prison. No wonder nightmares had dominated their sleep. And when they were in the throes of patient care, the injuries and death were so horrendous that their nightmares, by comparison, seemed child's play.

Bryson seemed intent on keeping the conversation light, asking W about his background, where he had gone to medical school, etc. Although the men had spent some time together off and on during the past several months, there hadn't been ample opportunity to hear details about each other's lives prior to arrival on the Continent.

Mary knew most of W's background, namely that he'd gone to Loyola, spoke five languages, and came from Polish immigrants. But as she listened to him talking to Bryson, it was as if she was hearing all of it for the first time. How could he express all his accomplishments without so much as a hint of arrogance? And he looked so handsome. Golly, he'd aged, but the marks of war had enhanced his good looks. W's haircut was perfect, his grooming always impeccable. How did the man have time to look so exquisite?

Then she began to appreciate the geometry of his face, the sculpted cheekbones and square jawline, his chin strong but not at all protruding. And his manner, his sense of decorum, she suddenly realized, were so much like her father's.

That she'd been able to hold back from succumbing to W's affections had been miraculous. There'd been moments during the past seven months when she had to rely on extreme discipline—the embraces they'd shared after losing a patient, the slight touch of his hand on her waist when he walked behind her in the wards, her fingers holding on to his when she sensed he needed forbearance to stop himself from going into some sort of tirade. Surgeons under stress could certainly throw a few, as Mary recalled later.

About 50 minutes into their trip, W felt Mary shivering. He asked Bryson to pull over so that he could pour the hot drinks. Bryson found a sun-drenched spot to stop the jeep. Mary wanted to dive into that sun and swim in it, she was so cold.

After hot chocolate, she finally warmed enough to ward off another series of rigors. But by then, they'd sat there too long. The sun's heat had melted the snow under the jeep's tires. Ice had formed around them. They weren't able to gain traction.

"Shit," Bryson said, as he killed the engine and jumped from the jeep.

W joined Bryson to take a look at the back tires. Both concluded it was hopeless to get the vehicle to quit spinning. And the jeep didn't house a winch on the front grille. Their only prayer was that an Allied "deuce and a half" would happen upon them and pull them out of the mess.

It was around two o'clock that afternoon before one appeared.

Bryson hailed it down. Within 15 minutes a corporal had wrapped the winch's cable around the steel bar that had been welded to the jeep's front bumper, a feature added to jeeps to defend against decapitation wires that the Germans had strung across Normandy's roads.

Now a decision would have to be made. Should they turn around and head back to command post or head to St. Hubert. They looked behind them and saw snow clouds fiercely accumulating. In the direction of St. Hubert, it looked only partly cloudy. Bryson concluded that they were much closer to the building they wanted to inspect than they were to Virton. The better choice was to press on with their original plan if Bryson was truly certain that they were that close.

Soon they arrived at the building and found it occupied with upwards of 200 children, most of them orphans. The sight of those beautiful, dispossessed children overcame Mona and Mary. After months of holding back any emotion at all, Mona lost her composure, her sobbing inconsolable, just like the night in the ambulance back last summer. As a result, it took far longer to tour the building than Bryson and W had gauged.

By the time they climbed back in the jeep it was less than an hour before dusk. St. Hubert didn't look promising as a hostel. So little was left of the town. They would have to head back to Virton as fast as they dared push the jeep. W said that they would just have to beat the snowstorm, but the tone of his voice didn't hold much conviction.

Mona made a mental note to look for any suitable shelter along their route just in case. She noticed a barn with tank tracks leading to its front opening. She knew they wouldn't make it back before dark, and already the winds had begun to push against the jeep, suggesting that heavy snowfall was imminent. Heavy cloud formations overwhelmed the sunshine the four had enjoyed earlier that day. Within minutes, even the few rays that had been determined to break through the clouds succumbed, and natural light was all but extinguished.

Bryson seemed to be the only one of the four who began to worry about another real threat other than the weather. Despite the impending storm, shelling from enemy aircraft was a possibility, especially since St. Hubert had been clear of clouds when they left it. If the weather there was still ideal, Luftwaffe could come from that direction, strafing until the clouds drove them back to their base.

In less than five minutes, his fear was realized. There it was—the familiar sound—the tat-a-tat-tat of the bullets popping against the road behind them, the plane's eerie Doppler sounds zooming over them.

Bryson remained calm and disciplined himself not to swerve the jeep off the road. He estimated that the four had enough time to exit the jeep and take cover in the ditch before the plane circled and took to shooting at the road again. And there was a slight hope that the strafing had been indiscriminate or had been a last hurrah before the ensuing darkness compelled the pilot to direct the plane back to his base.

The four hopped from the jeep. Mary and Mona scrambled like mice building a frantic nest as they were intent on carrying the green army blankets with them to the ditch. They crouched and fiddled with the blankets until they'd succeeded in covering their four heads. Bryson thought such an activity was ridiculous, blankets not exactly the ideal armor against machine gun fire. But he realized that Mona and Mary were past the point of employing logic.

The raging storm that had prevented their making it back to post had also dissuaded the Junkers Ju 87 from returning. But the light for that day had been extinguished. Darkness fell over them like a heavy cloak.

CHAPTER 26

KAR 98

Mary and Mona whispered to the men about their prospects of surviving the night. They couldn't chance driving the rest of the way back to Virton; their jeep having gotten stuck in ice earlier in the day had been a harbinger. It was too risky to chance it. If they wrecked it on the way back to post they'd freeze to death. And they certainly couldn't remain huddled in the ditch. The temperature was dropping too rapidly. They needed shelter.

Mona remembered the barn. It couldn't be more than a mile behind them, maybe less.

Bryson wondered if she had recalled tank tracks anywhere near the barn's vicinity.

She said yes. She was sure there had been tracks. They looked like they led to a barn door entrance.

Bryson knew that tracks were imperative. Without them, there was too much risk that the enemy could have planted mines all around a shelter like a barn.

Tanks were used to detonate personnel mines so that infantry could walk safely within the confines of a tank's tracks. Of course, teller mines had the capability of blowing the tracks off a tank, so if Mona hadn't seen any abandoned tank, Bryson decided the barn was probably their best option for shelter. He would go alone to check out the barn, and he'd have to make good time before the heavy snowfall camouflaged the tank tracks that Mona thought were there. He armed himself with a pistol, a flashlight, and two packs of Camel cigarettes. Mona, Mary and W huddled in the ditch with nothing to do but shiver and pray for Bryson's safe return.

During his trek to the barn, Bryson admonished himself for ever having gotten the four into such a mess. He felt that if it were up to him, he should be stripped of his major's rank. After a few moments of self-loathing, he decided that he better begin acting like a major again and devise a plan for surviving the circumstances that he'd put them in.

If he arrived at the structure safely, his next challenge would be to sweep it for enemies potentially holed up. Of course, if there were any Germans, Bryson knew he was a dead man since the only weapon he had on him was his pistol. If the barn was unoccupied, he would note its shape, check out how many entrances it had, and pay attention to whether the barn housed any or enough hay to provide warmth to the four.

If Mona had been right, then he should make it to the barn in just under 15 minutes. He checked his watch many times to approximate when he should begin looking for tank tracks. At 12 minutes into his trek, he pointed the flashlight down to peruse the ground. No tracks yet. At 13 minutes, nothing; 14, still no tracks. There wasn't a choice. He had to keep looking and decided that at 25 minutes, he'd head back and look again. Maybe it was further than Mona had thought, or maybe she was wrong and there weren't any tracks. At 17 minutes, he saw them. He walked gingerly, certain to keep his boots within the tracks' grooves.

He found the large barn door slightly open. He dropped to his knees to listen. The snow was now very heavy, but he had to make sure he wouldn't be leading his friends into a death trap if any enemy was inside. After about 10 minutes of complete quiet, he had to chance it and enter the structure.

There were two barn doors, one on the east side where he'd entered, and one on the opposing west end. There was hay, lots of it. Hurriedly he looked for a ladder, located one, and decided to get back to his friends with as much energy as he could muster. None of them had consumed lunch or supper. His lack of fuel reminded him to make sure to get each of the four to carry their canteens, and hopefully they hadn't drunk all the water he'd packed in the jeep.

Bryson went back for Mona, Mary, and W. They gathered all the canteens and the blankets and reached the barn without incident. Mary and Mona felt relieved, but Bryson told them that they had much work to do before bedding down for the night. He instructed the nurses to gather as much loose hay as they could and bring it to W and Bryson at the west end of the barn. Bryson figured that if unwanted visitors were to enter, they wouldn't arrive before daylight, and, if so, since the snow had stopped by the time the four of them had traversed to the barn, surely, they would notice the Americans' well-worn boot prints frozen within the tank tracks. Hopefully they'd follow the boots' prints and enter through the east door. Based on such an assumption, Bryson decided that he and W would build a hay shelter on the opposing side of the barn in a corner on the west side, far away from the more likely entrance an enemy might breach.

As Mona and Mary scavenged for loose hay, the men began stacking the few bales that were still tied together with ropes. The remainder of the hay was loose and would have to be piled as compactly as possible on top of the solid squares. Bryson and W formed two hay walls in the shape of an upside-down "l." They stacked one hay wall so that its end pressed against the western wall of the barn. Then they built the second hay wall adjacent to the barn's southern wall, forming a squared fortress. When the men had reached as high as they could, Bryson scaled the ladder and W handed him more hay to pile higher. They agreed that the walls ideally should reach about eight feet high if the gals could find enough hay.

But Mary ran toward them, harried and breathless.

She and Mona had found a wounded German boy. He'd covered himself halfway with hay before he'd fallen unconscious. Mona was watching him.

Bryson quickly descended the ladder and followed Mary and W. On the way, he asked Mary if the German was armed. She hadn't thought to check. He was unconscious anyway, but Bryson said that she was used to seeing patients after they'd been relieved of their weapons before arriving at the evac. She hadn't thought of that, but she had a decent visual memory. She thought he may have some sort of rifle with a strap, but she was sure he was nearly dead. She could swear her life on it.

They reached Mona and the boy. He'd hidden in the northwest side of the barn. Bryson figured that he had either entered the barn and made cover while Bryson had gone back to the jeep, or he was there all along and Bryson hadn't done a thorough-enough sweep.

The strap held a Kar 98 rifle.

Relieving him of that as well as any others that he might have on him was the major's job.

W knelt at the boy's head and felt his carotid artery, then lifted the top half of his body so Bryson could remove the rifle and search him for other weapons. There was a pistol, but it was unloaded.

The Kar 98 contained a strip, five bullets. W laid the boy back down and said he had a chance if they could get the bleeding stopped. His only injury seemed to be a gunshot wound to the right shoulder.

"Is he in shock?" Bryson asked.

Mona said she didn't think he'd lost enough blood to be in hypovolemic shock.

W agreed, adding that he was more than likely starving and dehydrated before he suffered the bullet wound.

Bryson surmised but chose to keep to himself that there was little likelihood that the soldier was alone. Possibly he'd been hit with friendly fire when the four of them had been strafed at dusk that day. If he had friends, they'd probably come looking for him at first light, if not before.

Bryson handed the Kar 98 to Mona while Mary ran back to their new hay hostel and grabbed one of her blankets for the men to use as a makeshift gurney. They dragged him about 50 feet to the southwest corner and placed him inside the newly constructed hay room, and Mona covered him with another blanket. He moaned a bit but never seemed fully conscious.

W used his pocketknife to tear off some of the German's sleeve and use it as a compression tourniquet to stem the blood loss. The poor kid didn't look a day over 16. They took turns watching him as the others gathered more hay and then attempted rest. Clinically, all they could do for the boy was keep him warm and stop the bleeding. The bullet must have missed hitting any major arteries; otherwise, he would have bled out by that time.

W looked at Bryson as if he also guessed that the boys' comrades might come looking for him soon. The men asked Mona and Mary to sit tight and watch the boy every second. They exited a small opening they'd made in the hay and discussed a plan.

First, they decided to use most of the scrap wood they could find in an attempt to form a barricade at the western door, the one just a few feet from their hay room. If the enemy were to breach the entrance closer to them, they needed to buy time with a barrier. Once that was accomplished, they used the few boards left to bar the eastern door, the more likely entrance if anyone were to follow the tank tracks. Since the eastern door was about 100 feet from their hay shelter, Bryson would have time to scale the ladder in the corner of the hay room and take shots at any enemy using the German rifle that he now wore round his chest. For the ladder to be secure enough to hold the stocky 170-pound soldier, he and W had been forced to prop it against the barn's wooden wall. The hay wall that faced the eastern entry wouldn't support him. Somehow Bryson would have to maintain his balance on the ladder from an insecure sideways position, with the right side of his body leaning against the southern barn wall. It wasn't ideal, but it was the only way that Bryson could have an advantage for shooting at potential enemy intruders before they had time to find his friends.

If any Germans chose to breach the more likely eastern entrance, the Americans would hear them coming and would have a fighting chance to scurry out a small exit they could create within their hay room. This would be their final task before settling on a schedule for watching the soldier and taking turns for sleep. They used pocketknives' tips to poke holes in two of the planks at the southwest corner of their square hostel and succeeded in creating a rough, zig-zag breach in the barn wall. Then they patched the escape hatch with hay.

Mona wanted to know if anyone had thought to bring water, whiskey, anything.

Bryson had, of course. But that was it. They had one canteen of water for what was now five of them, although the German was still unconscious, so he didn't count yet as far as water consumption went.

Mona and Mary lay next to the boy who had stirred only once when W and Bryson had placed him on the ground. The men had tied his hands with rope from one of the hay bales. No one could trust a Jerry, not even this one they were trying to save.

Bryson and W urged Mary and Mona to try to sleep. It was 2:30 a.m. by then. Daylight would be upon them in four hours. Bryson would take the first watch. W should get some shuteye, too, since the surgeon had been awake 36 hours. W didn't argue, but he urged Bryson to wake him at 5:00 a.m. so that Bryson could get one hour of rest before attempting to devise a safe way to return to the jeep.

They shut down the three flashlights in their possession and took a vow of silence. Sleep refused them for at least another hour, but finally W napped once he heard the soft purring of the two nurses.

At 5:00, W popped open his eyes. His mind had reminded him that his buddy Bryson needed rest. W insisted on keeping watch. Bryson resisted but decided that W was probably right. He did need a little rest just to be able to think clearly for the day's decisions.

At 6:15 a.m., Mary woke to check the boy's vital signs. He had made it through the night. Before she found the time to force herself into another coherent thought, her hands and upper torso bristled—there were German voices—she was sure of it—audible enough for her to know there were two, maybe three of them. It took the enemy less than 20 seconds to break through the flimsy makeshift stronghold at the expected eastern entry.

Bryson heard them, too. He put his hand over Mona's mouth and nudged her to wake. W stuffed a handkerchief in the boy's mouth, and stealthily scaled the ladder. He reached the eighth of 10 rungs when he secured a view of the enemy. There were two of them. There was no way to mask the noise that the bolt-action rifle would make when he cocked it. He had to shoot quickly, cock again and shoot a second time. Of course, the Germans recognized the distinct cocking sound of the rifle, but the major's marksmanship didn't fail him. He shot and killed them both within six seconds.

Mona, Mary, and W had tunneled through the escape they had created through the barn wall. But as soon as Bryson knew that he'd stopped the two intruders, he realized that he'd missed at least two possible scenarios that could happen outside the barn. The escape hatch led to the open field, not the tank tracks. The three could inadvertently set off a mine in their attempts to escape. And what if the intruders had left other comrades to sweep the barn's exterior? He'd given W his pistol, but that wouldn't be enough to defend against more enemy soldiers outside if they were armed with rifles. Because of these horrific possibilities racing through his head, Bryson wanted to get to his friends as quickly as possible. He attempted to jump from the eighth rung of the ladder, but before he could secure his left foot to the rung, his boot caught underneath it and caused him to lose his balance. He fell to the ground on his left side, fracturing his left ankle.

CHAPTER 27

Blue 88

With his belly on the ground Bryson pulled himself to the opening of the escape hatch his friends had exited not three or four minutes before. He saw them in the distance and cried out to them to stop, but they couldn't hear him. They were mindlessly floundering about in the deep snow in the open field. He knew that he'd be forced to get them to stop. He propped his body against the southern exterior of the barn wall and searched with a predator's eyes for any enemy. Seeing none, he cocked the rifle again and shot in the air.

The three couldn't help it. They had to turn back to look toward the shot's sound. When they saw him, it was as if they all immediately understood what they had just done, stunned with the reality that they may have just run through a minefield. Mary fell to her knees and wept.

She remained on her knees and began thinking of Robby. If she had been maimed or killed by a personnel mine, or by one of the Germans she'd heard in the barn, what would Robby have thought? Why was she away from her unit? What was she doing in that field?

W bent down and attempted to console her. Mona stood completely still, knowing not to take one more untested step, and stared blankly across the field toward Bryson. He called out that it would be okay. They should return to the barn but re-trace their steps exactly.

It took them a while. They couldn't make a mistake. Finally, they reached the barn and crawled flat on their stomachs back through the escape hatch. W assessed Bryson's injury. He wouldn't be able to walk without some kind of aid, and now it seemed too risky to move again in daylight. More Germans could be close by. They spent the rest of the day figuring out what their next move should be.

The two boys that Bryson had killed were armed with rifles, each with one full unused strip of bullets. So that was 10. The Major had shot three of the five bullets from the strip that had belonged to their patient. That meant they had a total of 12 bullets. But only Bryson and W knew how to shoot rifles.

At that point they figured the 39th was probably packed up and ready to move out of Virton. Maybe the evac's convoy would happen upon their abandoned jeep, or maybe someone had noticed by now that the four of them weren't back from having checked out the school at St. Hubert. Mary said that she'd told Alabama that they were going, but Alabama was going to work the night shift, so she may still not have had a chance to even question where Mary could be.

Mona had told no one, and W had secured a 48-hour leave. He began thinking about what he'd said to the acting chief nurse. It might be a possibility that since Mona and Mary weren't expected to be on duty for 48 hours, she may not have missed them yet, either.

What was their better option, Mona wanted to know. Should they go to Virton? What if everyone had left already for St. Hubert?

W speculated that there should still be a skeleton crew in Virton like there always was after most of the unit moved on to a new post. Critical patients were always held back until stable enough to travel.

W whittled down some of the shards of wood left over from tearing the hole for the escape hatch. Mary cut strips of cloth from the two dead Germans' uniforms to use as ties around a wood splint for Bryson.

Mona continued to check the German boy's vital signs. They'd kept him warm. They'd stopped the bleeding. It was time to attempt to wake him and try to get water down him.

Their water was almost gone, so each of them reached through the escape hole and stuffed snow into their canteens. Melted dirty snow was better than no water at all. The hay room rose above freezing that day, thanks to a prolific sun that shone all afternoon.

By 2:00 p.m., though, Mary had been so thirsty she'd drunk too much of the dirty snow and began vomiting. She was now of no use to anyone and was furious with herself. Now they'd have three patients to take care of, but W couldn't tend to her. It wasn't plausible for all four to stay there again that night. Bryson needed either surgery or casting soon or he could end up with a life-long debilitating injury if that bone wasn't set. They didn't want to split their team, but if more enemy soldiers showed up they would have to face that whoever was in that barn, whether it was two of them, or four, there was a big possibility that all would be killed. Two should go at nightfall and at least get the chance to return to the evac. And it had to be W and Bryson. Mary was sick, and Mona didn't have the strength to hold Bryson up for the trek back to the jeep. Only W was strong enough. If they got lucky and guessed correctly, that the unit probably was still in Virton, they wouldn't have far to drive. They recalled that they were approximately 50 minutes into their road trip when they'd been strafed the night before. That meant that Virton was no more than 12 or so miles away. If the 39th had not finished packing for St. Hubert, then W could see that Bryson got immediate treatment and then could secure an ambulance. W would ride back with the medics at first light the next morning to help them locate the barn.

The men would leave the barn at dark through the eastern door. Earlier that day, W strapped one of the Kar 98s round his chest to defend himself against any enemy stragglers before venturing out to re-trace the tank tracks. He used the longest piece of scrap wood he could find to deepen one of the tank tracks again for his and Bryson's use come nightfall.

Through a second night holed up in the barn, Mary and Mona would remain with the German who was now coming in and out of consciousness. Of course, it had crossed Bryson's mind to simply "leave the Kraut," send an ambulance for him once all four returned together to the 39th. After all, he'd killed two of the boy's buddies that morning already. But he knew that he was up against three caregivers who wouldn't have considered leaving the boy. Besides, there was the other dreaded possibility that he and W could be caught by the enemy as they attempted to get back to the jeep. Again, it was better for two to be caught than all four of them.

This night wasn't as black as the previous one with its cloud coverage, but the barn wasn't more than 50 or 60 yards from the woods that lined the road. During the afternoon, Bryson had practiced his new gait with the splint securing his left ankle, but he couldn't walk on his own. The splint helped, but there was too much risk that he'd fall and suffer more fractures. If he was in pain, he was far too heroic to mention it. He calculated that he and W wouldn't be out in the open for more than 20 minutes "tops" because his friends had done a remarkable job make-shifting a splint for him.

The four walked to the eastern entry of the barn. Mary hugged W and stuffed a Hershey bar in his coat that she'd just thought to look for. Her vomiting had ceased, but she couldn't hold any water down, clean or dirty. W promised that an ambulance would be back for them at first light.

In the last few moments, nobody said anything. There was one more round of hugs, and then they were gone, leaving Mary and Mona alone with the German boy.

They returned to the hay hostel and Mary checked on the boy. He was so still that Mary thought that he might have died in the few minutes that they had taken to say goodbye to W and Bryson. Something about the possibility of that young man's death caused her to begin shivering. They'd been through so much for this boy. And earlier they'd gotten about six ounces of water down him, and W had said that if the ambulance were able to reach the barn within the next eight to 12 hours, the boy had a chance.

His pulse was elevated, but that was to be expected.

"Oh, thank God," she mumbled, and then her teeth began a methodical chatter. Mona said that she sounded like a metronome set at about 180 bpm.

The hay room's temperature had dropped significantly since the sun had abandoned them. But it wasn't only the freezing hovel that caused Mary's audible shivering. Her body's dehydration had set her on a perilous path. She knew it. Mona knew it.

There was some hope. They trusted that W and Bryson would make it back to post. The German boy might have a chance. W had said so. She and Mona weren't dead yet. And the patient seemed to be enjoying a deep, wondrous sleep. She envied him as she hovered above him like a doomed helicopter.

Mona piled hay as high as she could in one corner of the hay room and forced Mary to crawl into the space. There was one blanket left to share. The boy had one underneath him, one over him, and the dead boys shared the third.

Mona faced a clinical dilemma. She could coax Mary into drinking more of the dirty snow water that had made her so sick, but Mary would probably refuse. Or she could wait until Mary was almost asleep and then wake her when she was in a semi-conscious state and trick her into taking in the water. That might be the better option.

She shivered, too, but she knew her shivering had more to do with her fear than her body temperature. But they were in a place where fear and cold were indistinguishable.

The fear was rooted in facts that she had to face. Because of one stupid decision to travel to St. Hubert there was a chance that she would lose her three best friends in one night. Bryson and W might be doomed somewhere between the barn and Virton.

She couldn't control what might be happening with Bryson and W. She forced herself to focus on the fact that was right in front of her. Mary was falling away. Why?

She began laying out the facts. Mary's pulse was elevated, 130 bpm. And she was purring, probably in deep sleep, which meant that her resting heart rate should have been only 65 or 70 bpm at most.

Then it hit her.

Mary hadn't been vomiting all day because of the dirty snow water. After all, W, Bryson, and she had been drinking that water all day. They hadn't gotten sick. She'd mentioned earlier that her mouth felt like it was stuffed with cotton. She'd said her body ached all over. She was so lightheaded that she looked as if her swooning was going to cause her to fall on top of the boy. And now her pulse was so high. Jesus. Mary had been vomiting because she was symptomatic of severe dehydration. Both W and Mona had missed it clinically.

"Shit," Mona muttered.

Her anguish stretched the hours. There was so little that she could do other than pray that W got Bryson to treatment and could stealthily grab an ambulance before anyone knew it was gone. She tried to do the math. If they'd been right about the approximate distance between the barn and Virton, and if W were to leave at first light, it would put him back there in four hours. But then she forced herself to ask what could be the longest amount of time it might take for W to get back to the barn with help. What were the potential obstacles? The unit—everyone might have left for St. Hubert already. The weather—for all she knew another snowstorm could be brewing. The medics—who could W trust to keep their mouths shut about the entire situation? Thank God Chief Maxson wasn't there.

At 4:00 a.m. Mona got desperate. Mary's heart rate was too high. She was close to hypovolemia. At 3:00 she'd contemplated the idea but told herself to re-visit it in an hour. The hour was here. The thought had been to try to slow down Mary's heartrate. Try to buy Mary some time to prevent organ failure. It had occurred to Mona at 3:00 a.m. that maybe she should put a Blue 88 in Mary's mouth. She had some. One of the paratrooper patients had given a few to Mona a couple of months ago. Was it risky to give Mary one? Yes. Administering a barbiturate in a severely dehydrated patient. Was that the thing to do? What if it made her worse? It shouldn't, though. It should help her body maintain more moisture, shouldn't it? She thought it should. Whatever volume Mary had left, Mona had to preserve it until the ambulance got there. It might be Mary's only chance. Her rapid heartrate needed a slowdown. And maybe the German boy needed one, too. Maybe she should put a Blue 88 on each of their tongues. But what if this killed them? What if she was wrong? They only gave Blue 88s to soldiers to calm them. What if it slowed Mary's heart rate down too much? She would have killed her dearest friend. But if she didn't give one to her? Could Mary last until W got back?

At 4:10 a.m. she put a Blue 88 on the tongue of the boy. She'd check his pulse at 4:30. She had no guilt about using the boy as her experiment for Mary's sake. At 4:30 a.m. he was still alive. His pulse rate had slowed. Now for Mary.[1]

1   Interview, Lorraine Matzke, Spokane, WA, 1978.

CHAPTER 28

For the Boys

Paramount in Mary's mind was why they were there. She asked Mona, but Mona wouldn't answer. Mona wasn't listening. Mona was stubborn. She just kept saying to rest, to calm down. But Mary didn't want to be calm. She wanted Mona to answer her. She wanted to know why they were so cold.

At least her annoying thirst was gone. That starving for water and not having any was so hard. Earlier she'd imagined canteens full of water, delicious, fresh mountain spring water. Thousands of canteens full of it in her mind. She'd salivated from the image. But now she didn't really care. Thirst had left.

But that swimming feeling. She was so dizzy. She was sort of drowning, but it was like she was drowning in a dry cloud. Strange. A dry cloud. Like a cloud full of sand, not water. She wanted to get back to thinking of why she and Mona were here. It felt important to go back to that.

Those boys at Pearl. That's why she was here, maybe. But what was it? Grief? Yes. It was that awful grief. She couldn't oblige that grief. It hurt so bad. It was too heavy. That grief for the boys, the boys at Pearl. That horrible time they brought in Redmond. God, Redmond.

And all the boys whose hands she'd held, pretending to be their mother when they were dying. She'd lied to them. She'd let them call her "mommy," "mama," "mum," "*Mutter*."

But what else? Why was she here? Mona didn't answer her. Then Mona said something. She said something, but Mona seemed far away, and Mary couldn't hear her. What did she say?

Fight. Mona said fight. It was just too hard to fight. Mona didn't understand. Everything was just too sad. Too much. Mona said to get mad. Throw a fit, Mary. Get mad that we're here, Mary. That's what Mona's saying. But why are we here, Mona? Why?

For the boys, Mary. We're here for the boys, don't you know?

Just before leaving consciousness there was a thin thread of awareness surrounding what Mona was asking of her. Mona wanted her to find what she'd felt when she'd heard about the boys at Pearl. Mona wanted Mary to find rage again, however distant and elusive.

CHAPTER 29

Lucky Strikes and a Limey

Belgium
January 31, 1945
Dearest Family,

> Guess I told you we moved again and have been very busy. Last night never stopped once except fifteen minutes for chow. Right now, we're waiting for the next load. My eyes sure get tired at night, as there is so much book work and the lights are poor, and the generator is screwy half the time. The first part of the evening I was working by flashlight. This time we're set up in a former boys' reformatory which has been hit so there are boards on all the windows, but our quarters are fairly comfortable now—the only inconvenience being that we carry wood and coal and pails of water upstairs all the time, but we're used to that by now.
>
> I went on a scavenger hunt the other day and got two pails and a nice wash basin and two chairs all of which were buried in the snow which is quite deep here now. On my way back to quarters I sat in the wash pan and slid down a nice little hill. I didn't think anyone was looking but, of course, about six GIs came along about that time, and boy was my face red. Gee, I've been getting lonesome for my skis, but even if I did have them, it wouldn't be safe around here with unexploded mines and booby traps, which the snow makes more treacherous.[1]

She hadn't written home in 15 days. When she finally did, she chose to remind them, and perhaps herself, about her youthful days of snow-skiing, of simpler, more innocent times. No need to worry them about the harrowing days in that barn.

W and Bryson had no scares along their journey that night, save that they couldn't get the jeep cranked at first. They made it back to Virton and found the 39th still there. W consulted with a surgeon who'd specialized in

---

1   "Booby traps" was a term loosely used by nurses to refer to any enemy-planted device. In most cases, they were referring to land mines, which, in military terms, was incorrect. The military definition of booby traps specifically referred to detonators that the enemy often placed in deceased bodies or which were hidden among the ruins of towns.

orthopedics back in the States, and Bryson was admitted. X-rays revealed that W had been right about Bryson's fracture. The orthopedist ordered a sedative and set the bone.

W found Poncho, who told him that much of the unit was set to leave the next day at first light, and they would convoy to St. Hubert by borrowing some vehicles from other evacuation units nearby. Poncho helped W arrange transport back to the barn by borrowing two EMs from the 101st Evacuation Hospital and one of that unit's ambulances. W gathered medical supplies.

They reached the barn within 30 minutes of leaving Virton at daylight. They brought along water and food. The medics checked vitals on the German boy and then loaded the dead boys in the ambulance and placed the corpses on the road so another ambulance charged with picking up the dead would spot them and see to it that they were dealt with appropriately. Then they drove the ambulance back and loaded the boy, still alive, and Mary, also still alive; however, both patients had fallen into unconsciousness. Mona told W what she'd done. She'd gone through with it. Not only had she given the German boy a Blue 88, but at 5:00 a.m. she'd put the little blue pill on Mary's tongue. She'd taken a huge risk. W relieved Mona's mind. By God, he'd said, that was smart.

He'd been able to employ his smarts, too, despite his anxiety over having left Mary and Mona so vulnerable to the cold and possibly having abandoned them to be killed by an enemy that knew it had lost the war, for all intents and purposes, and therefore would have no reason to keep Mary and Mona alive. He had forced himself to overcome the stressors of these possibilities long enough to employ the doctor within and brought along several IVs of fluid, assuming that Mona and Mary would also be dehydrated. This turned out to be the best decision he could have made. Mona would be given it prophylactically, Mary and the boy emergently.

An advance team with some clinical support had arrived in St. Hubert the day before, so the ambulance headed there. W rode in front with an EM. The other medic managed the German boy in the back.

Poncho located himself to his rightful place in the world, beside Mary in the back of the ambulance. On reaching St. Hubert, Mary's condition improved dramatically after having been given the IV drip. Within two hours she was cognizant and teasing Poncho. Apparently, Alabama had tried to give him a crew cut when she was a bit inebriated. Poncho had decided the best route after such a disastrous outcome was simple—he shaved his head and was complaining to Mary that it was "cold as a witch's tit" in the back of that ambulance since all his hair was now gone.

During Mary's mere three-hour hospital stay, Poncho stayed with her and kept her entertained during the administration of the bolus of fluids. He scooped her on the latest scuttlebutt and included important information, too. Apparently, General Patton had made it clear to his top brass to remind their divisions, units, platoons, etc., that much work was still to be done. Hitler was still alive, demanding that his troops maintain strongholds in every German town between Prum and Berlin.

> February 2, 1945
> Dearest Mom,
>   … Our next move will undoubtedly be in tents again. There just aren't enough buildings left standing as we head north. People are getting optimistic about the European Theatre again, but the awful feeling we had a few weeks ago is still too vivid in my mind. Well, even if it does end soon there are many of us who will have to go to the other theatre and, golly, Mother, I'd do anything to get out of that. Robby will probably have to go. I don't know. Anyway, all we can do is live from day to day and keep dreaming and hoping and praying. And I'm really praying for Robby these days. You know probably that things are coming to a head again over here and after the sights we've witnessed during the past few months, but it's not something I dare tell you about…

W and other physicians met with Major Scanlon who forewarned them about the types of injuries they were to see when Third Army troops began perilous river crossings necessary to drive the enemy back toward the Rhineland. Many Allied boys drowned in the flooded Moselle River, and Mary walked around so sad for days when she was told that one of the lieutenants she had known since Fort Leonard Wood had been one of the Moselle's victims. But a couple of days later, hope sprung eternal when that same officer showed up at the 39th to say hello to Mary. There were hugs of great relief when he told her that he hadn't been anywhere near the Moselle.

On February 7, however, TUSA troops were facing an even more deadly river crossing. Third Army lost about 60 men who attempted to cross the Sauer's rapid currents. In other areas the Sauer's waters flooded its banks, disguising the barbed wire that went along the Siegfried Line.[2] Soldiers became tangled in the mass of hidden wire.

Colonel Bracher became increasingly frustrated when his unit couldn't keep up with Patton's rapidly advancing troops. Sometimes there just weren't any

---

2   The Siegfried Line, marked with pillboxes, tank traps, and other fortifications, was formed along the western border of Germany. Used in World War I, it was re-fortified and added to during the years between world wars. Germans commonly referred to it as the "Western Wall," but for the most part it was not effective. The line of fortifications looked like dragon's teeth, reminiscent of the Greek legend.

suitable buildings left. Other times his recon team would return from having secured a suitable location only to find out that SHAEF had promised it to another unit. During these times the 39th would be relegated to treating non-combat injuries.

Mary was assigned what she called the "Shock Ward," and she decided that it was the most difficult place in their hospital to nurse. One day she took care of a poor "Limey" who was admitted to the ward after having been a prisoner of war for five years:

> When he was first captured, he was only twenty years old. And now the poor kid's 25. He's lost most of his teeth and has a hydrothorax, but you should see him. The boy's so positive, and ever since the psychiatrist told him that he can go back to England soon, he's walking around smiling like he has the most gorgeous set of teeth in the world. But then, all of a sudden, he forgets that he's not a PW anymore and starts spitting out fluent German. Golly, the boy just breaks my heart when I hear him doing that.

After having taken care of the Limey, she wrapped herself into her sleeping bag and then sat up on the edge of her cot, sharing a Lucky Strike with Alabama.

Alabama handed her the cigarette again. Mary declined it, saying that she had a sudden headache and that maybe cigarettes don't agree with her.

"Well, then stop smokin' 'em. And I'll smoke for both of us. They don't give me a headache. Just this god-awful war does."

She and Mona still hadn't told Alabama about their perilous days in the barn, and they swore they never would; however, the light duty day found the three of them holed up in their third-story bombed-out dorm room in the former boys' school. Soon they chatted the way they used to at the Buckley house. Mary brought nuts and brownies that she'd gotten from the Red Cross set-up, and they'd take turns removing themselves from their sleeping bags to stoke the fire's wood and coals.

Alabama hadn't been fooled. She knew they were gone. She'd cut Bryson's hair that day, so she figured that the four had double-dated to only God knows where afterwards since she never saw hide nor hair of any one of them for the rest of that day and the next. She poured champagne to loosen Mary's lips while Mona took her turn to stoke the coals.

Mary's voice quivered when she recounted their decision to press on to St. Hubert after having been pulled back onto the road with the winch. That was their big mistake, as hindsight had come to them as early as that first night in the ditch. They'd lamented to each other that they should have returned to Virton earlier that day instead of sticking with their original plan to head to St. Hubert. She re-hashed most details of the subsequent events very accurately, according to Mona, who crawled back into her sleeping bag and muttered an affirmative tone during each break Mary took to sip more champagne.

Mona took over the telling when Mary reached the part of the barn's sequence of events on the second night. Naturally, Mary didn't remember most of that night.

No one ever really knew why Mary had reached such a severe state of dehydration when the other three had not. Probably she'd begun the trip dehydrated and didn't know it. And cold weather can mask a person's ability to recognize a need for water.

Alabama said that Mary probably sweated too much despite the cold because Mary always tended to overdress. She was always so terrified of the cold that it was her habit to layer too heavily which could cause sweating and, therefore, a loss in water volume from the body.

There were probably many physiological reasons, but the clinical outcome was the only one that mattered. She'd made it. Mona had made it. Bryson's bone was healing. And W was still very much in love with Mary. But that was a problem to be solved a different day.

For now, Alabama drew out her long arms from under her sleeping bag and pressed Mona's head on one of her shoulders and Mary's head on her other one. She said something that Mary never forgot.

"Well, looks like you're gonna become old women 'spite the fact that you've been tryin' to do everything in your power not to get there. Sorry, ladies, you're gonna get old and ugly, and I hope I'm there right along with ya."

CHAPTER 30

Luxembourg

They weren't sure what cities were being bombed. They'd heard that the U.S. planes took care of most bombing raids during the day, and for the past couple of months on clear weather days, they'd seen them, like multitudes of flying, roaring lions, with mythical fat wings and what looked like massive turds dropping out of the beasts. "Turds of death," Poncho called them.

On February 10, in St. Hubert, it took Mary and Mona all night to shower and launder. They walked up a steep, muddy hill to the showers, and then they dragged water upstairs to wash their clothes and kept the fire going in order to heat the water. Mary had learned not to allow her laundry to pile up because it was simply too burdensome to do so. On their trek down the hill after their showers the two gals boasted about the fact that they noticed they never got sick like they used to, that they must have become immune to exposing their wet heads to freezing temperatures. The days of complaining about the hardships associated with living outdoors or in shelled-out buildings were over, it didn't seem to faze Mary anymore. In fact, she said that she rather enjoyed the challenge.

It turned out to be a special day for Mona. When they got back from the showers, she learned that she would receive her silver bars and first lieutenant rank. Mary wrote of Mona's promotion, "I'm so happy about it. If anyone ever deserved it, she certainly does."

On February 19, Mary, Mona, Alabama, and many of the nurses who had served in the 39th since their arrival on the Continent on July 19, 1944, were issued two new bars to wear on their sleeve, each one denoting six months of overseas service. By then they had earned four battle stars, representing four major campaigns. Mary was particularly pleased that they all received a new battle dress each, as well as "several cute shirts and short jackets." They relished the knowledge that Uncle Sam had begun awarding them for their service and loved feeling feminine again in the new uniforms.

But by the end of February, Mary noticed that Mona's depression seemed to have returned; worsened, she guessed, by the prospect that it might be months before Mona would see Bryson again. He was back at war, and notwithstanding the few moments she'd laughed with Alabama, she'd gone back to that shell-shock pallor she had during that ambulance ride to Arrou. Compounding her depression was the fact that the 39th's rapid movements to support the troops would eventually take them back to living in tents. Mary found herself giving Mona emotional support by making sure that Mona always had a fire, even if she had to use her bare hands to dig through mounds of burned-up coal and ashes to get it started. She took it upon herself to do *anything* to help Mona get through that difficult spring.

> March 6, 1945
> Dearest Daddy,
> ... I could write a book on the scenes we witnessed on the way up here (Vianden, Luxembourg). Of course, we passed through what's left of Bastogne and every town from then on—they were all ghost towns. The wrecked tanks, planes, vehicles, dead horses and cattle along the roadside detracted from the beautiful country. We are so high it seems like we could reach out and touch the planes as they go over. About a five-minute walk from here we can look at the dragon's teeth and pillboxes of the Siegfried Line...
> Did I tell you that Paul Ferreira, our Transportation Officer and Robby's friend, got us some celery from Brussels? It was the first we'd eaten since we've been overseas...

She decided that the letter to her father needed to express joy over something, but a stalk of celery? Good grief. When she read over her words, as terrible as her description was of the ghost towns and the dead horses, she had intentionally chosen a laconic path, keeping details to a bare minimum.

The convoy circled and trundled through Bastogne and on toward Luxembourg. Along their route, night fires entranced them, and the memory of them would never leave any of them for as long as they lived.

The Royal Air Force flew the night sorties. The fires east of them looked like they were reaching as far as the Rhineland. Someone muttered that by the time the 39th reached Germany, there might not *be* a Rhineland.

What in God's name had the Germans brought on themselves? The fires looked close. As far as they could see, there were pockets of fireballs and waves of flames. The entire continent east of the Ruhr River seemed to be burning, and yet, everybody felt stone cold.

Then came their arrival in Luxembourg. Mary couldn't write the truth about it, not even in her diary. Words had lost the ability to resolve the images. They'd be with her the remainder of her life.

It was dawn. W, Mary, Mona, and Dagny had taken an ambulance as transport from St. Hubert to Vianden, Luxembourg during the wee hours. They'd been told that the 39th would set up the hospital in a former sanatorium. Major Scanlon and a crew of enlisted men were ahead of them, but when the major saw the conditions, he turned his jeep around and headed back to stop the clinical personnel before they arrived. The major asked them to get out of the ambulance. Although confused, they obliged him.

The six of them and the ambulance driver stood on top of the hill adjacent to the hill that would be their new home. On the hill on which the sanatorium stood, hundreds lay dead, some incinerated, most charred, all unburied. As soon as the stench hit their nostrils, the onlookers vomited in unison.

Major Scanlon asked them to remain there. "Just sit tight," he said, until he could gather enough enlisted boys to clear the hill of the dead. Mary adored Major Scanlon, particularly because he maintained a thoughtful, calm presence at all times. The dead of Vianden, though, slaughtered, burned alive, abandoned without proper burial—that experience changed him. He looked twice his age in a matter of minutes. He got back in his jeep and headed toward the task at hand.

W tried to get everyone back in the ambulance, but some of them felt too sick to their stomachs to get in the vehicle at that moment. They needed fresh air, but there wasn't any. The breeze touching their faces was saturated with a putrid, noxious gas. And then they all began to feel guilty. There was something depraved, vile, about vomiting. To respond with regurgitation seemed the height of disrespect for the dead on that hill, but the taste of the dead in their mouths didn't oblige their guilt.

Then W muttered that it was just like his nightmare.

Mary knew what he meant. He'd told her about a dream that had haunted him—he, Mary, and others, standing together on a hill, cold, even though they could see fires that seemed to reach as high as the stars. Then there was a pristine village, like a scene from a Renoir painting, then that same village, burned up, with charred figures entombed from the ravages of a desperate and savage time.

Deposed Queens

One happy moment stood out during their time in Vianden. At the sanatorium's makeshift mail room, Sgt. Parent combed through boxes and letters. He came across a ship-by-proxy parcel addressed to Mary Balster and immediately knew its contents.

He found Mary working in Medical. The package was tiny, just like the engagement ring inside it. Robby had come through. His sister Minnie had chosen it and had sent it from the States. In big cursive letters she'd written, "Congratulations, Mary. We are all anxiously waiting to meet you. Take care of yourself, Minnie."

It was a perfect fit and everyone, including W, noticed her newly adorned ring finger.

They weren't posted at the sanatorium in Luxembourg for long, and the 39th had never been happier to close camp.

The nurses couldn't have been more pleased with their next post. Col. Bracher was able to secure the 39th to headquarter in the Adolf Hitler Kaserne (Barracks) in Bad Kreuznach, Germany. All agreed that it was "the nicest set-up" they ever had, a complete reversal from their Vianden days.

There was evidence that some German officers and their families had lived there before the Allied forces drove them out. Mary, Mona, and Alabama stole furniture out of the attic and the basement. They fixed up their rooms with the remnants the Germans had left behind, and the girls played a game imagining that they were decorating their own homes stateside.

Alabama announced that they were actually "livin' somewhat like real queens" or in the least, "like deposed queens."

> The girls in the room next door have a radio which is playing beautiful, dreamy American music. It makes me so lonesome for Robby. And yesterday was his 27th birthday. I feel like crying, but that just isn't done anymore.

It's probably broadcasting some German program designed to tear down our American morale. They do that all the time, you know, especially one program in which "Sally," a German girl, speaks English and plays Bing Crosby tunes—all designed to make us homesick. Of course, everyone knows the fake Sally now, and we all just laugh about it. But the music, admittedly, does get to us.

The 39th's advance across Belgium, Luxembourg, and now Germany had offered little chance for W and Mary to talk. And the intimacy had been sparse. A kiss in the dark after a long shift before someone walked by, a friendly hug on the occasion that they ran into each other after chow, his hand across the flank of her back as he walked behind her, that particular expression of intimacy Alabama had noticed months before.

W had been asked to consult on some patients hospitalized in Belgium just after the 39th took up residence at the Adolf Hitler Kaserne. But before the unit was moved again, he returned.

Wearing the engagement ring had been so much more enjoyable when W was in Belgium but became burdensome upon his return. Mary decided the better choice was to simply avoid him. But there was no way that he was going to accept the ducking. At midnight, a nurse across the hall tapped on Mary's door and said she was needed downstairs.

W was waiting for her in the living area. He'd found a quiet place for them to talk.

It was the dining hall of the Adolf Hitler Kaserne. It gave them a creepy feeling to think that the Third Reich had dined and planned horrific scenarios in that same room, so he handed a Camel to Mary.

She took a long, deep drag and said that she really was not at all keen on Camels anymore. She was sure that they were causing nasty headaches. He asked her if she'd prefer a Chesterfield. They weren't as strong.

But they stuck to Camels and talked for over an hour. He'd been aware of her habit of choosing angst rather than hurt anybody's feelings, male or female. A lot of women tend toward such an exigency, but Mary's was extreme. She'd always choose others' feelings over her own. She'd sacrifice any of her own needs and paid too much homage to loyalty to past promises, regardless of present circumstances or changes in her life that she couldn't have predicted at the time she made those promises. He wondered if she even recognized the gal that she used to be on that ship bound for Liverpool, the gal who fell in love with Robby.

She avoided answering the Robby question but admitted that she had numerous faults. And certainly, most of the people who knew her were quite willing to make a list for her, lest she forgot any.

He hadn't asked her to come down to the dining hall in the middle of the night to add to the list. He was simply suggesting that she just might be happier if she let go of the past, stopped trying to control everyone else's thoughts about her. He reached for her hands across the table, held them with a firm grip. Had she ever really forced herself to ask why she made certain decisions and, if so, did those decisions align with what she really wanted? Or was she sticking to decisions because her mother had practically threatened to disown her if she didn't keep her engagement promise to Robby? If she didn't want to take an honest look into her reasons for maintaining her engagement, it may end up haunting her. He was older, had seen people make that mistake, people who had refused to ask themselves why they made certain choices and then later realized the choices led to outcomes they weren't expecting, outcomes they wished they could change. He wasn't criticizing her. He didn't consider her allegiance to others to be a "fault," as she had described it. He only wanted her to consider her own needs and quit the little-girl antics of always wanting to please her mother.

She sat across from him chain smoking the Camels and took an abrupt turn from her impulsive nature. Instead of immediately answering him, she asked him to stop with the questions, allow her some time to think.

He told her that was "in and of itself an improvement," that he was happy to see her quiet herself.

She took the next five or so minutes to remain quiet, lost in her own thoughts. She didn't agree with anything he'd said. Life was much more haphazard than that. It took you where it wanted, no matter the plan you had in your head. Take the war, for example. She wanted to serve her country. She hadn't planned on the fact that her service would cause her to fear for all those she loved every waking moment. And if that weren't enough, sleep was no guarantee of a break from that worry and was usually wrecked by horrifying nightmares, some even less horrifying than what they'd often experienced. And yet, despite the hell of the past several months, what incredible rewards signing up for service had led her to experience. She'd saved Redmond, maybe hundreds more, held others' hands to award them a little peace by pretending to be their mother. She'd fallen in love with Robby, had forged lifelong friendships. She'd been shot at, survived the mine field. And to top all that off, she'd found out what it meant to be so hungry and wet and cold with Mona in that barn, but as miserable as she was, she still fought to survive the experience. She understood why some might choose death over that level of misery and fear. But always she chose life even though she had no idea how it would pay her back the next day. It might still turn on her and leave her lifeless on some unknown, vacuous hill. Still, she believed that it had all been for some reason that she didn't understand. All she knew was that she hadn't planned any of it. But the spectacular misery of it all had produced in her a joy that she never would have been able to plan or create out of her own volition.

And as far as her deserving anything good, that wasn't a matter of speculation. She knew that she didn't deserve anything good. Look at all the boys and gals who had died. They didn't deserve that. Their families didn't deserve to feel sad for the rest of their lives. She was no better than any of them. Yes, she'd always fight for survival, but there would always be guilt. There was no way around it. Guilt was the thing she'd already packed—if she made it back home.

They meandered back to the kitchen to find snacks. W convinced her that the headaches probably were related to her chronic hypoglycemia rather than from smoking. She didn't have a great record of taking care of herself.

The neoclassical kitchen stacked white tiles with black grout, stretching six feet up the walls from the chessboard-patterned black and white floor. The tiles bordered sterile, white plastered walls that met a 12-foot ceiling. Three chandeliers overhung a long, curved stainless steel counter. Along the back wall, white marble countertops still held a few statues typical of neoclassical design and left from the Third Reich's days. One was of an eagle spreading its wings. The vast and harsh space carried the same kind of chill one gets the first time the sharp breeze of winter moves through the body.

The center counter's sheet of steel gleamed under the chandeliers, shining clean from the proud work of the 39th's kitchen staff. The last of two from the cleaning crew were leaving when the captain and lieutenant walked in, but not before giving them a tour. Of course, the doctor captain and Lt. Mary could help themselves to anything. One of the PFCs lit an eye on the massive stovetop and placed a kettle of water for tea if they wished. The other showed them the bounty of food that the last of the Germans had left behind.

There were jars of nuts, breadsticks, fresh butter in the cooler, cheeses, olives, Coca-Colas, and German chocolates. W and Mary stuffed themselves silly. In addition, the chef had been able to procure some sugar rations and had baked a German chocolate cake. At first, she said no to the cake, but W stuffed a piece in her mouth. Before she knew it, she'd gulped a big slice and chased it down with a cup of hot tea. He knew how to brew tea the only way that Mary could drink it—strong. It was the finest tea she'd ever had, and she uttered a soft thank you.

W's physical presence had held Mary in a heightened state for months. But in the kitchen, in the wee hours of morning, his every move overwhelmed her. She hadn't been drinking, but she felt drunk, dizzy. Maybe something was in the tea.

Now the black and white kitchen didn't feel stark. All at once, she felt warm. Her face flushed. W moved toward her. He touched her cheek and then bent to kiss it. Taking her hand, he led her to a pantry off the kitchen. It was dim and small, but somehow cooler. As their eyes adjusted to the lack of light, they discovered the shape of the room. It was round, almost like a ball turret. There was a draft of cold air, too cold for Mary. A window had been left half open. He told Mary to sit, but there wasn't a chair. He laughed and asked her what was wrong with sitting on the floor. After all, she'd been sleeping on the ground for the better part of two years.

While W shut the window, she found the only wall that didn't house shelves, slid down it, and sat. Then he sat next to her and extinguished the light from his cigarette. He pulled her small back toward him and kissed her face and then her mouth with an intensity that didn't seem as if it could possibly last. There wasn't any way that anyone could kiss like this forever. These kisses didn't feel as if they belonged in this world. The longing, the urgency, the messages from the kisses were ones that he couldn't possibly have meant to send. They were respectful but fierce, penetrating. Now he was a hunter with intense, purposeful, black eyes, controlled and controlling, in charge and not willing to yield. There was a look of respect but there was also a look of dominance, of calculated supremacy. How could such a predator make her feel what she was almost sure she was feeling—trust? He brandished every movement of his body. He was premeditated, a Roman warrior. How could he look so calculating but so reckless? His untamed kisses, his arms, like lassos, entangled her, pressed her down, insisted that her shoulders lie flat against the floor, pushed her into a compliance but with the loving strength of Atlas. Then he moved his hands to her torso, then her legs, compelling them to lie obediently flat and still. He pressed his chest against hers. A dizzying series of throbs pulsed in her head. A heaviness moved over her body. Her breathing felt different, calmer.

There was in her a strange dichotomy between thoughts of feeling safe versus thoughts that some outside force must have descended on them. Was it a force of corruption? And if so, why did it feel so enticing? Why did there seem to be in her a need to throw away the rules she'd set up for her life? Was this mere instinct? Or was this something beyond intuition, beyond anything that she understood as reality?

Somehow, the moments drew her back to those images of the supply room on the night she defied the rules to save Redmond. Was this act of allowing

DEPOSED QUEENS • 195

W the privilege to touch her also an act of defiance? But this time an act of defiance to save herself? Was she going to allow herself to turn away from the mantra she'd lived by for the past year? Was she destroying the future she'd planned with Robby? Or was she saving herself?

There seemed to be some sort of rapturous force overwhelming her. She wasn't in control. It was so strong it easily devoured her own resolution. Now she had no recognition of any of the words that she'd said to W less than an hour ago. None of those words seemed genuine now. They couldn't have come from her mouth. The only truth right now was one that seemed to exist outside of her, something that took over her and negated the story she'd been telling herself for a year.

In place of words, or logic, or mantras, there was only this—a drunken onslaught of swirling and tingling that began to crush and then defeat any remaining forces of inhibition that may have been left in her. An incessant and tidal rush of tiny explosions rippled through her. These ripples of seemingly untouchable places ached for invasion. They demanded their own surrender by insisting that this man cover every inch of her body with his physical power, wrap her in savagery. The clamoring explosions fired in rapid succession, the ripples continued to ignite, rise, fall, the ups and downs of their demands to be extinguished only by a pristine, pronounced, palpable intrusion. They demanded their own execution. They wanted to be gripped, shoved, tugged, corrupted. They wouldn't stop their insistence that the bliss they brought was nothing compared to the utter violation of their own destruction. They wouldn't stop their terrible billowing until that heavy, bombarding cascade, that fierce and violating barrage, pounded them into submission.

The light allowed by a clear dawn angled through the small window and lit her eyes. It looked to Mary as if he were searching her eyes to make sure that she was surrendering. She tried to mimic the insistent and penetrating kisses he was giving her. She wanted him to understand that what had been before didn't matter to her now. Tomorrow didn't matter, either. Finally, she wanted to show him her willingness to surrender to the heavy bombardment of his exquisite power.

Nevertheless, she would make him work for the right of the invasion. She didn't protest, but she wasn't willing to help him. She dropped her hands along her sides to allow his removal of the brown and white seersucker. There wasn't anything now that was going to be able to fight the complete and utter longing of him to descend, raid, foray.

She knew that all these months, his longing to take her had been quelled by the impact of war and patient care. There'd been no time to connect with her the way he'd wanted. There'd been his signals, his hand on the small of her back when no one was around, the gifts he'd brought her from Paris, his continual search for somewhere, sometime, some opportunity to satisfy his longing for her.

Maybe earlier that night, his insistence that she begin to try to figure out what she wanted rather than always choosing others' wishes over her own, maybe that had had an effect. This submission to him—wasn't she indicating that she was willing to try on the idea to live and choose for herself? Did this open, genuine act of surrender hold an irony? Through letting go, wasn't she showing contradictory proof of making a choice for herself?

Later that night, he said that she wasn't like his previous lovers. When they first met, he said that he'd been smitten with attraction for a girl nurse named Mary. But after having seen her sacrifice her physical and emotional health repeatedly during the last several months, a woman had been born.

The only sign of girlhood left was the brown and white seersucker, tossed aside in a rumpled disarray of defeat.

CHAPTER 32

Buchenwald

Two days later, the 39th moved to Bad Hersfeld, Germany, and as sorry as Mary felt for herself for loving two men, she felt twice as sad for Mona. They would be back in tents. Mona fell apart when she found out. If only she could hear from Bryson, that he was okay, then perhaps she could withstand the tents again.

On their first day of their hospital opening there, the rains were intolerable. They hadn't seen that much mud since Tennessee maneuvers. But the days they spent in Hersfeld were not without amusement. All the nurses were fond of their newfound penchant for gathering trinkets, discarded pots and pans and other household items formerly owned by the enemy. One of the items Mary cherished the most was a full-length mirror. Although it was becoming cumbersome to cart such rubbish around every time the 39th moved, the girls managed by rolling up most of their treasures in their bedrolls.

By April 7, Mary and Mona had organized their tent, having rummaged through a house on a hill vacated by German officers. Down the hill and into the tent they dragged furniture and straw mats, the latter to serve as flooring. The ground was still so damp and cold. The engineers had outfitted their abode with a little coal stove, the smoke of which went through a pipe that extended up and through the tent's top. Mary perched the new mirror against one of the tent's side walls and crept onto her cot and into her sleeping bag.

Just as she had settled herself, a frigid wind with gusts exceeding 40 miles an hour howled and pushed like a monster at play.

> Just a little while ago I was sitting on my cot reading and writing letters and all of a sudden, the big mirror fell as a result of a God-awful wind gust. The top of it crashed into the stove pipe. I had to run out of the tent but fast to keep from dying of smoke inhalation. So much for being a vagabond. Mona was upset because some of our stuff burned up and the rest now smells like coal dust.

During the second week of April 1945 General Patton moved TUSA Headquarters from Frankfurt to Hersfeld and had two trailers parked adjacent to Mary and Mona's tent. They'd seen him a few times during the fall of 1944, but in those days, Mary avoided running into Patton. She wasn't at all confident with her salute technique at the time and had told Poncho that she would choose death by spontaneous combustion over receiving an admonishment from General Patton. But by April 10, 1945, Mary owned a crisp salute and a GI attitude. It was thrilling to see him, and she made it a habit to watch for him and his entourage when he took his morning walk.

The general encouraged every member of the evacuation hospitals attached to his army to visit the Buchenwald concentration camp. As much as Mary admired General Patton, she couldn't bring herself to go. She wrote to her parents that she had seen enough death and destruction for many lifetimes and that she was certain their "famous general was wanting to make sure that everyone understood why we must not end the fight too soon, that we still had much work to do to decimate and crush the enemy, even if it took thousands more American lives to accomplish it."

She recalled her angry period during the November before, how she had said that "our boys were getting killed and maimed" for no reason. Now she fully understood the reason, so she didn't feel that it was necessary to be reminded. She still hadn't gotten over the sight of that hill in Vianden. No Buchenwald for her.

Some of the boys of the 39th Evac had grown so tired of army rations they decided that, while the patients had been doing their part to defeat the enemy, they could do theirs and kill a cow. On April 21, they treated the entire 39th—personnel and patients alike. They were the best darn steaks they ever had.

> May 6, 1945
> Dearest Mother and Daddy,
>   Well, it really looks as though things are about to wind up over here; however, we are still very busy with battle casualties...
>   Daddy, thank you for enclosing that excellent article detailing how patients are cared for in a Shock Ward. It's a most authentic description concerning a nurse's duties on that type of ward. I've been in charge of Shock Ward many times during the past several months and, undoubtedly, it is the most depressing, smelliest, and most backbreaking place in the hospital, but what a wonderful feeling to see a patient at death's door come back to life.
>   When I've watched patients die, I've so often thought whether I should write to their folks and tell them about their courageous son, but one never knows how people will feel about those things. So often they ask for their parents, especially, of course, for their mothers, and I've held many a boy's hand and pretended I was his mother at the end. I always say to them something like "better you should sleep. Everything will be okay when

you wake up. Rest." And most of the time I've been lucky, and they close their eyes and die, thinking their mother's right there with them...

Now the roads are lined with millions of down-trodden Germans. They seem to be lost—some in uniform—the rest in ragged clothes traveling in everything from ox-drawn carts to trailers and wagons or anything they can obtain. Much of the time the women are walking while the men ride and there are more children than I've ever seen in my life. It all looks like a big mess and will take years to straighten out. How the U.S. is going to feed all these people beats me...

CHAPTER 33

Hopes Unrealized

VE Day (Victory in Europe) officially came on May 8, 1945. By that time only the 39th and one other evacuation hospital remained attached to Third Army. Two days later it was announced that the 39th would soon act as a station hospital as opposed to a semi-mobile one. Now that the fighting was over, the field and evacuation hospital set-ups were no longer appropriate for patient care. The 39th would be attached to fixed buildings somewhere in Germany, although they weren't promised when. Although the war was over, to be in a real fixed hospital again still seemed to be the "stuff of dreams," Mary said later.

Germany
May 10, 1945
Dearest Family,

Just a few lines before I crawl in my sack again. No matter how early I get to bed 0600 always gets here too early. Dissipated a bit last nite and didn't get to bed until midnite must be getting old as have been tired all day today.

It's hard to believe that V-E Day finally arrived. Can't get used to the fact that we don't have to worry about the Jerry planes at nite, buzz bombs, not wearing helmets, and so very many other things. It just doesn't seem possible but how very wonderful it is.

We are still terribly busy, however, all NBC's [non-battle casualties], but as there aren't any Gen. Hosp. set up in the Rhineland, we are getting everything and have been especially busy treating the allied liberated prisoners. Have everything on our wards from Poles, Russians, Czechs, French, and Limeys and of course our own wonderful GI's. You wouldn't believe the stories they have to tell, but the evidence is all here that all that they say is the truth and also from what we have seen. There is nothing but bitter hatred in our hearts for our crushed enemy and nothing can be too bad for them. I hope the army of occupation will not relent and lose that feeling—if they do, they will be traitors in my estimation because they will be betraying those who have died for this cause. For so long I thought what in the world are we fighting for, but in the last month have definitely decided that we were all fully justified in fighting this war and any trials that we have endured are so very small compared to our boys.

We will be moving shortly to act as a station hospital for a while and sweat out either the boat home or to the CBI [China Burma India Theater of War, the War in the Pacific]. Here's hoping it's the former—everyone thinks they're going to be the lucky ones to go home, but in our hearts we all know that many of us won't for some time. Do think, however, that Evacs have a better chance of getting home, but please don't get your hopes too high at least for a couple months. Rumor has it that we are going to move into buildings very close to Switzerland. Sounds like a good deal so far and hope we're not disappointed.

Received the wonderful cookies, candy, and shower slippers and once again thanks a million, and the girls send their thanks too.

The sun finally came out for V-E Day and has shone warm and bright ever since. Can hardly wait until my bathing suit arrives now so I can get a coat of tan… ETO mail gets worse every day and of course I'm always fuming about that because I miss Robby's letters so darned much but then they usually come in a bunch and then I'm always relieved to know that he's writing most every day. Received a very sweet letter from his sis in Columbus, Miss., the one who selected my ring. Her letters are so typically southern I can almost hear her talk. Sure hope Robby and I get together before we get much further apart, although the distance between us is at least 400 miles. We are barely inside Germany—in fact just about 10 miles from Czechoslovakia.

Guess I'll put a quick end to this as I'm awfully sleepy. Until next time so long for now and heaps of love from your army nurse.

Mary

VE Day didn't bring the desired relief that the 39th and all those who served in the ETO had imagined. During April, everyone focused on comparing his/her Adjusted Service Rating (ASR) scores. The decision as to whether a soldier would be sent stateside for leave or would be ordered to serve in either occupied Germany or the war still raging in the Pacific was largely dependent on that soldier's ASR score.

In a letter Mary received from Robby in late May, he mentioned that his ASR score was high so it looked like there was no way he would be going to the CBI first. He would be awarded extended leave stateside. And if somehow the Allies were to defeat Japan while Robby was back in the States, then he planned to leave active service and head to El Paso where his friend Harold Womack had secured him employment in the hardware business.

Despite her noted skills as a nurse, Mary's disdain for army authority had never waned. Consequently, she held one of the lowest ASR scores in the 39th. It was so low that she still hadn't been promoted from her rank as a second lieutenant.

Have had some lovely patients in this area and they have paid me some very high compliments for my nursing, and all insist they are going to write to the general to see that I get a silver bar. But they don't understand that it's not the way a nurse treats her patients in the army but rather how many apples she can polish, if she's strictly GI and gets everything down on paper so it looks good to the brass that really counts. I don't say that many who have their silver bars aren't worthy because they certainly are but it's just like anything else in life, I guess. It doesn't matter two hoots to me whether I ever get one—have always considered my first duty to be the welfare of my patients and to the best of my knowledge I have a perfectly clear conscience on that score. As to violating uniform regulations, coming in a little late, or being caught eating on the ward and not saluting the right people—well... really 10 years from now it won't make a bit of difference...

The May 1945 letters held an irritable tone. After all, she was living with the knowledge that both Robby and W would be going home and that, barring some miracle, she would not be, given her underwhelming ASR score. She was now paying the price for all the times she had been remiss to follow army rules and regulations. A substantial list of infractions had been mounting since maneuver days when she and Lorraine had committed many. And getting kicked out of the Buckley billet in Altrincham didn't help her. She was quick to run to Chief Maxson to take the blame for that debacle, always protective of Mona's stellar reputation. In Mary's mind, Derek was to blame for it, but since Derek wasn't in the ANC, all the blame was placed on Mary and, as she now surmised, placed in her record. She hadn't realized that her conduct was continually being counted toward an ASR score. Mary never thought in those terms because she knew how much the army needed her skills. And her devotion to patient care was never in question.

Certainly, that letter of commendation that Chief Maxson promised her would have helped elevate Mary's abysmal ASR score. Unfortunately, as fate would have it, Maxson never returned to her desk duties in the 39th after that awful ambulance wreck. Consequently, Mary's letter of commendation was never added to her military record.

She always figured that her skills, along with her German fluency, would hold her in good enough stead to prevent her from receiving a dishonorable discharge. Of course, she was right about that, but her inability to follow the rules, especially during the first year and a half of service, was finally catching up to her. She might very well end up having to pay a massive price by being ordered to the CBI. And if this wasn't enough, the 39th's living conditions had deteriorated again:

This period we are going thru now is a million times worse than the adjustment period in England and at least we were living in comfort then but now here we are stuck in this stinky and I mean really stinky cow pasture as the odors which rise from the ground around here are nauseating (too many closed latrines and dead buried in them). Anyway, we're stuck with not a blessed thing to do which I never could stand anyway and just waiting and waiting. The Munich trip turned out to be another unrealized dream, so I guess we'll just stay in these blasted tents until we go home or elsewhere. The mud and rain we've had all week doesn't help our spirits any… please, please don't ever have a bean in the house when I come home or any corned beef, or I'll capitulate on the spot. And if I ever hear that song "No Letter Today" again I'll break the radio…

We've been reading every bit of print we can lay our hands on to keep from going nuts. During the past week have read *Random Harvest, Dragonwyck*, and *Also the Hills*, good books all of them, but you can't live in a story book world with grim reality staring you in the face the rest of the time.

Twenty nurses are going home next month—some of them to stay, others on leave but I'm not one of them and Mona is, and some of my other best friends since Maneuver days. If we don't get leaves then I'm just going to the Colonel and beg for one to go see Robby as he can't come into Germany according to the rules. Of course, I'll probably be refused as he won't let us out of his sight. The other nite we were invited to a lovely party given by some officers in a division in this area. It was in the most gorgeous, modern building I've seen in Europe. These Germans were so far beyond any other country when it came to modern conveniences but then of course they robbed the other countries to do it. Anyway, the floors were covered with beautiful thick rugs. There was a chromium horseshoe bar and the latrine fascinated us—you pressed a button and two sliding doors opened into a mirrored room and when you stepped inside the cubicles the lights went on. The division had their orchestra which was super, and we danced on a paneled floor of dark and light wood which was as smooth as glass and the most handsome American men in the world—everyone in pinks and blouses and all wearing their numerous battle decorations. There wasn't too much liquor but every kind in the books including champagne which is my favorite, but we didn't waste time drinking, and we did everything from jitterbug to tangoes, and rhumbas… Anyway, my friend took me home in his jeep but as he decided not to take his driver and comes from a long way from here, he didn't know the way and we got lost and it took us an hour to get home. I sure got razzed when I got back, but I told everybody it wasn't that we wanted to take the long way home, as it was pouring rain and a jeep is little protection in inclement weather, and I never wanted to get back so bad in all my life—even to a cold, damp tent…

By May 30, there was no doubt in Mary's mind that she was in for at least five consecutive years of service before she'd be allowed to return to the States. If she married Robby in Europe, she'd be given leave for a honeymoon as an honorably discharged officer's wife, but that leave would be followed by a return to service either in occupied Germany or in the Pacific Theater:

Tomorrow, we start an intensive training program so better I should get caught up with my correspondence today. Our training program will include everything we did in England for 5 months except this time we will study diseases pertinent to the CBI. According to the reports this theatre was child's play compared to that one as far as living conditions are concerned. But there is no use to dwell on the future, and we can only take things in their stride and make the best of them. By this time, we are quite used to making some pretty rugged adjustments and no matter what comes am sure we can cope with it. I don't live in the future anymore because that seems to cause more heartache than living from day to day and all we can do is try to find some happiness in each day…

We were just reminded that today is the day we are to think about and pay our respects to our honored dead by several very loud reports from some kind of weapon shooting red, white and blue rockets into the air. Now the band is playing "The Star-Spangled Banner" which always sends chills up and down my spine. I never felt that way until we landed on foreign shores. The sight of the American flag is just as thrilling. Now the German women are making flags for the various units over here and they're very beautiful flags and what a wonderful feeling to know that we are Americans and have such a beautiful place to return to.

Her training, however, would have to wait. On June 1 she was admitted to the hospital for severe exhaustion and pneumonia.

Mary's internist admitted her to the hospital and charged Gladys Stinson with managing her care. Stinson was about 20 years older than Mary and had become one of Mary's favorite mentors. Soon, though, Stinson became exasperated with the number of visitors Mary was receiving and, although she didn't dare mention it to Captain W, she whispered to Mary that he was the worst offender of visitation rules and needed to quit "hovering" and allow Mary to rest. After Mary's third day in hospital, Stinson recommended to Mary's internist that Mary be discharged and placed under enforced bed rest with no visitors.

During her convalescence Mary finally received a letter from Robby. He was still stationed in France, but he didn't state his exact location. Even though they hadn't seen each other since December 10, 1944, his salutation always addressed her as "My Darling Wife."

Sweetheart, I have before me three wonderful letters that came yesterday and today. The one written the 13th of May and then one from the 15th and the 16th, so after a hard day I had something to look forward to. But in every letter, you had different information as to what your unit was to do.

In one you were to get three choices—is that out for good now? Gee, I was so in hopes you were to go home and do service in the States if you must stay in the Army. If you have any choice whatever, darling, be sure to take service at home. I certainly don't want you still over there if you can get back to the States.

Don't worry about me not seeing you, sweetheart. I will definitely be up there in a week or so. I must see you so I can talk to you about our getting married over here.

In one of your letters, you seemed to have the impression that I wanted to wait. Gee, of course honey it would be better if we waited but gee, I am so darn tired of waiting. Not that I wouldn't wait the rest of my life for you though, darling.

It's the waiting one has to do in the Army that is so darn hard.

So, your Dad advised against it, well honey, he is right, I know, but when we see one another we will definitely decide and make our plans accordingly.

Say kid, how is that sunburn you got? Gee, don't you know better than to get in the hot sun with a shot? Gee, the shot gives you fever to start with. You need me to be there and take care of you.

Golly, I wish you would have been here yesterday and could have taken care of me. Boy I was sure a sick G.I., but I managed to get up today and was O.K., except a little weak. Feel pretty good now though.

Received the nicest box from your mother yesterday. Gee, she is so darn sweet sending me things like that. Really, she shouldn't, though, for there isn't a thing I can send her…

Darling, wouldn't it be wonderful if we could be home together for our leave then get married and have a thirty-day honeymoon?

Well, Womack isn't back from the hospital yet. It looks like he will have a good chance of going home. I think he has stomach trouble—they're not sure yet.

Patterson made Major and sure was glad to see it, as he is such a good egg. Works pretty hard, too.

You don't have to ask me to forgive you for your griping, darling. Boy, I bet I gripe twice as much as you. Gee, what a Rebel's temper I have, and to just think that you've never seen me mad. But who could get mad at a girl like you? Gee, darling, what a wonderful personality you have.

Well, sweetheart, I am still just a little shaky so, if you don't mind, I will sign off for this time. Mary, darling, I love you with all my heart and miss you more and more each day.

Be sweet, darling.

Love always, Robby

She only got one letter off to Robby before he was there in person. Stinson had done some digging and found out that Robby had been moved to Nuremburg, so she sent word that Robby should visit. On June 18, he did. He bent over her cot and shoved his hands under her back to pull her towards him. All he could feel were bones.

But by July, thanks to her youth, Mary recovered fully. Robby remained stationed in Nuremberg, and Mary and Mona and the dwindling members of the 39th finally moved to a station hospital in Amberg:

The hospital is all white and shiny inside, and you know a military hospital is always a million times cleaner than a civilian hospital. It's really lovely—real hospital beds, telephones, elevators, beautiful sun porches, hot showers and bathtubs—everything a hospital should have and just the right size for our unit. I'm in charge of a messy ward (venereal patients) but like to work so much in a real hospital again (dressed in our seersucker dresses and caps) really don't mind it a bit.

Our nurses' home is darling—have three club rooms downstairs. Mona and I share a lovely room with cute wallpaper, bureau, wardrobe, buffet, etc. Our window looks out over the beautiful countryside as we are a couple miles outside of town, right in the country. We also have a super outdoor swimming pool between our home and the hospital. Our Mess Hall is also a dream—three dining rooms each with paintings and chandeliers. Have real white linen tablecloths and napkins with fresh flowers on every table, and German waiters wear white—the head waiter wears a tux.

Although their environs had become in their estimation luxurious, Mary continued to wrestle with the nagging prospect that any day she might receive orders to head to the CBI. Most of the ward boys, including Poncho, had already received their orders and were now all gone, some stateside, some to the Pacific.

To her great sorrow, Mona's orders to return to the States came soon after they'd set up their quarters in the room with the cute wallpaper. Mona had decided that she would remain in the service, but the army was awarding her some time with her family before she would receive her next army assignment. Mary couldn't even imagine choosing to remain in the army, and they laughed at the horrifying images of Mary as a career army nurse.

Alabama's orders were expected any day. Before the three were separated for the rest of their lives, Mary and Alabama sat up all night to help Mona pack. The three drank champagne and talked about the uncanny irony that it was Mary who would be the last of the three standing in the 39th, as they certainly knew of no one who had run the greatest risk of leaving so many times during the last two years. In fact, Mary became one of only eight nurses remaining in the 39th out of the original 48 who had boarded the HMS *Andes* bound for Liverpool in February 1944.

CHAPTER 34

The Green Danube

It was late July. Hills of verdure descended gracefully to the banks of the Danube. Parallel to the river ran an ashen roadbed so full of potholes that it reminded Mary of the time she and Lorraine had been tossed about in the back of the car that took them to their quarters that first night at Fort Leonard Wood.

W borrowed a jeep. He drove while Mary served as navigator, pointing out any future dip in the road that he should avoid. He'd planned for them to spend the day touring the Bavarian scenery. Behind Mary in the back seat was a Val-Pack loaded with tomato sandwiches, popcorn, two slices of German chocolate cake, and six Coca-Colas they'd stolen from one of the wards at the hospital in Amberg.

Their plan was to picnic on the grounds of one of about 20 medieval castles that had survived the ravages of two world wars. Mary had been curious to see the one that another nurse from the 39th had visited the Sunday before. She'd said that on the southeastern side of this castle there was a neglected rose garden that had managed to produce a voluminous display of fuchsia and blush pinks. Mary brought along a couple of old *Stars and Stripes* newspapers to wrap the roses in, just in case she and W could sneak about the garden and cut a few with his Swiss army knife.

Unlike virtually every day she'd spent in the army, this day went exactly as planned. They found the castle, the neglected garden, cut the most exquisite roses without anyone being the wiser, then threw down the OD blanket they'd brought along and ate a perfectly divine stolen lunch. Then they drank the contraband cokes while they gazed down at the Danube that was as green as the hill on which they perched. No blue in the Danube that day, although they considered it a marvelously pristine river all the same.

Mary had agreed to spend the day alone with W if he swore to not bother her about the future. He kept his promise to not argue with Mary about her decision to marry Robby. He did bring up the elopement plans, wondering if she and Robby were still planning to marry in Europe.

She had decided against elopement in Europe since the main reason for doing so had to do with the prospects that she would be sent to the CBI. As an officer's wife, at least she would be granted a leave back to the States before reporting for duty in the Pacific. But after the nuclear bombs were dropped over Hiroshima on August 6 and Nagasaki on August 9, she and Robby no longer had practical cause for eloping in Europe. With their worry that Mary's war service would be extended to the CBI now extinguished, they could take their time and decompress a bit. Robby was expecting his orders to return home any day. He planned to wind up his army service back in Mississippi, spend time with his family, then drive to St. Paul, perhaps in time for a Christmas wedding.

W said that despite the practical reason for eloping, he had gotten the distinct notion that Mary had not been all that enamored with the idea of elopement anyway.

Mary took her time to answer him and looked down at the roses that served as the centerpiece on the OD blanket. W had wrapped them up to their necks in the newspaper because he didn't want Mary to prick herself with the thorns. He said if he left the thorns on the blooms they would last longer.

She held her gaze on the pinks and, with a remarkably pensive tone, she finally answered him. His notion had been correct. She wasn't all that excited about eloping. At first, it sounded romantic. But soon after, she realized that if she chose to have some stranger walk her down the aisle instead of her own father, she would be choosing a vexatious sense of regret the rest of her life.

Had she not betrayed her father enough already by joining the war behind his back? To marry without H. C. giving her away, well, it would add more guilt to a list already too long.

She wondered if W thought there was always a price to be paid for perfect beauty. Germany, for example. Why the hell would the Third Reich go and ruin such a beautiful country? Why couldn't they leave well enough alone?

She was transfixed by the roses and rhetorically asked if they were not the choice metaphor for this thought, this truth that beauty can't exist without a lethal price. A rose's perfectly exquisite blooms can never exist without the accompanying thorns. Aren't they the most startling reminder that beauty can't exist without pain, without price, she asked.

He supposed she was right.

The afternoon dropped away. It dissolved into a swirl of summer days and evenings spent riding horses, dining in fine German homes now occupied by top brass, conversing with artists and musicians. Granted there were many times when grief struck each of them hard—when they were reminded of all the boys they had lost, all the innocents who'd perished because of the evil nature of greed and its consequence—war. Despite these unspeakable reminders, they managed to manufacture suns that dropped away into sparkling evenings in which Mary's most endearing characteristics, namely her beauty, charm, and spunk, captivated all those she encountered.

But one by one, the numbers of delightful people dwindled with orders arriving almost daily for each of them. By mid-September, W had received his and was back in Chicago. And Mary finally received confirmation that all Class 4 units were to be out of the ETO by the end of October.

She boarded a ship bound for the States on October 31, 1945, and by mid-November, she was back in St. Paul as a civilian.

CHAPTER 35

Isolation Has its Perks

Memory is a kind of consciousness, a sort of renewal...

WILLIAM CARLOS WILLIAMS

On November 15, 1945, Mary took to her bedroom at 1262 Stanford, and apart from two afternoons, she remained inside 1262 Stanford until February 24, 1946, the day before her wedding. Her family agonized over her self-isolation. Each tried their own tricks and pleadings to entice her out. She didn't mind too much if they visited in her bedroom, but no amount of coaxing resulted in her joining them downstairs for afternoon tea or for the munching of popcorn by the fireplace while listening to the radio's evening news report.

The bathroom was down the hall, which proved problematic at first. She ran the risk of running into a family member. So, she formed a habit of waiting until the copper pipes stopped clanking before she crept down the hall to the bathroom. There wasn't much competition for it anymore. Connie had married already, and most of the time Nancy was only home on some weekends from college in Madison. Still, one could never be sure of avoiding running into Inga or H. C. in the hallway, so better she waited until all inanimate sounds stopped, the ones that houses make during the night. Then she could shuffle in thick socks and oversized slippers to the steamy respite produced by the plentiful luxury of hot water and soft bubbles.

Her parents had given her an ultimatum. She could stay in that room until the end of February. They'd continue to coddle her with meals left in the hallway, but if she wasn't out by February 24, they'd have their good friend Boris knock down the door. Her wedding was slated for February 25, for God's sake.

At first, isolation had its perks. The first stage of isolation was enticingly luxurious. Wallowing in nothingness held such an allure. There was no present, no past. There was no pressure to take on the future. It was like being in a perpetual bubble bath where the water never gets cold.

There were no decisions to make. No time to get up. No time to go to bed. If one stayed in the bed all the time, then getting out of bed didn't even have to come up, other than for bath time.

She understood Mona now. Mona had it right. To separate facts from any emotion associated with those facts—now that was the way to get through things.

This plan worked especially well during the first phase of isolation, perfectly executed when Inga harangued about the darn wedding.

Was Mary planning to go to Chicago soon to pick out a wedding dress? Or did she want to just wear a suit? Many brides didn't feel right so soon after the war about wearing white. She'd read that in the paper. That was fine, but Mary needed to decide soon. There was always the chance that whatever she picked might need altering. God knows she'd probably lost more weight.

One of Inga's tricks succeeded in getting Mary to leave her room. She planned a reunion of some other nurses from St. Paul who had served in the war. That afternoon in December, Mary descended the stairs to greet the nurses for a lovely reunion, but as soon as they left, she thanked Inga for hosting and then retreated to her room.

And it was Inga who unwittingly forced Mary into the second phase of her isolation. She called out from the hallway, "Mary, it's December 20 already. You're just going to have to get some things decided."

December 20. It was a year ago to the day that Redmond was admitted with the tank injuries. Jesus. Why'd she have to say the date? Poor Mother. She didn't know. It wasn't her fault.

The date brought up the past. And the past had been securely buried during the first phase of isolation. Now it wouldn't stay away. Now everything in her room reminded her of them. The kid curlers—Mona. The scissors on the bureau—Alabama, the time Chiefee mentioned that Lt. O'Reilly needed to cut Mary's hair. The castle talisman stuffed in her nightstand drawer—Zim. The little tank—Robby, of course. The empty champagne flute—sweet Poncho. Daddy had left a silver tray in the hallway that held the champagne bottle and the flute. She grabbed the tray quickly and locked the door. Poncho had brought champagne to his three favorite lieutenants. He'd popped the cork in that field of bugs. Jesus, the necklace still hanging from the mirror—Clinton had given it to her.

Sometime in January 1946, she had an epiphany. Maybe not an epiphany but at least, finally, she had an answer to the question Mona had angrily shouted at her after the Derek Buckley debacle. Why on earth did Mary have such a problem with letting go of people who were no longer in her life? Why did she pile them up and never let them go?

She knew now. She couldn't let anyone go because then they'd become someone she used to know. If she said goodbye to Clinton, to Zim, to Lorraine, to Poncho, to W, to Alabama, to Mona, then they would become ghosts. And if she always ended up saying goodbye, if she let them go, then, at the end of her life, wouldn't everybody just end up being someone she used to know? They would all just become ghosts. That wasn't bearable.

There was only one choice. She couldn't leave that room until she figured out a way to deal with the ghosts. They didn't belong to her anymore. Mona was right. To truly love them, she couldn't leave them piled up in case she needed them later. That wasn't fair. They deserved to be dealt with. Somehow, she'd have to get them to a place safe in her mind where they could live but be free of her, and she could be free of them.

CHAPTER 36

Winter Storm Brewing

Mary felt safe to descend to the kitchen when she knew no one else was at home. As she pilfered in the refrigerator, the kitchen phone rang. She answered it, expecting a call from Robby. But the call was from W. He wanted to drop by, just for a brief visit.

She told him that he couldn't. Inga had been spending an inordinate amount of time at home watching her like a damn hawk. She wouldn't take to the idea of his visiting 1262. He said that he wasn't afraid of her mother. She knew that, of course, but Inga scared the shit out of her.

So, he suggested that they meet at St. Paul's Cathedral. Could she possibly be there by 1:00 that afternoon, he asked. By that time, the sun might get a chance to burn through the heavy clouds so surely full of snow.

For once, Mary was on time. Unbeknownst to W, it was the first afternoon that she left 1262 since returning from the ETO three months before.

She needed to get warm, so they found a side door into the cathedral. She hadn't been able to gain any weight. She was forever cold. They found a small sofa in the great hallway that led to the sanctuary. They sat for a short time, didn't talk about anything remotely unsafe. Certainly, he knew better than to ask her anything about Robby, although he did ask her what day the wedding was to be.

Other mundane conversation rounded out their short visit. Soon he stood up and handed her the gloves from the floor. She hadn't realized that she'd dropped them. Then he bent over, kissed the top of her head and her right cheek.

He'd better hurry back to Chicago, since it looked like a winter storm was brewing. On the way to the door, he looked back at her. She was still sitting on the sofa. He was wondering if she recalled that time on the Danube when they'd stolen those roses.

Yes, she remembered. He'd been thinking about that conversation, how she'd gotten it exactly right about beauty not being able to exist without something always around trying to ruin it.

Funny. She'd been thinking about that a lot, too.

He opened the door and met a brisk and sharp winter wind. Would she do him a favor? He was hoping that she could keep him somewhere in that mind of hers, keep him in some place that didn't ever go away.

He didn't have to worry about that, she said. He was already there.

Afterword

Mary held fast to the graces and decorum of her youth. I helped her to the recliner in her upstairs bedroom. When she sat, the tips of her toes barely touched the carpet, her posture much like a ballerina's. She never had thought much of any gal who slumped.

She crossed her knees, bent over to peel off the high heels, then said she was a bit loopy from the champagne and needed to take a little nap. She was always cold, so I found one of the afghans that Inga had crocheted. I think it was the green and black one. I helped her recline and then followed her instructions to cover her up "to the chin." She asked me for her slippers. They had possibly disappeared under the bed. On the bedstand was that red volume of war letters. I teased her, asking if she was re-reading what she'd written about a hundred years ago.

Family lore had it that she'd danced with General Omar Bradley one time and that she'd known General Patton personally. Admittedly, I never believed a word of the war stories, but then again, I'd never *read* a word of them, either.

I wanted to know if the stories were true. She said that it was just a funny little thing, the dance with Bradley. She and a girlfriend from the unit had been awarded a weekend pass post VE Day. They decided to go to the French Riviera and pretend to be two French gals. They got by with faking their French girl personas at a dance in which most attendees were GIs who didn't know French anyway. A few male officers from the 39th were there as well when General Bradley approached and asked her for a dance.

Immediately she was conflicted. Should she hold to the pact made with her girlfriend that, no matter what, they would both keep up the French gal façade all night? Or should she allow herself five minutes with the general to be herself because she sure was itching to talk to him? She chose the former, but consequently all she could say to General Bradley was "*oui, oui*." At the dance's conclusion, Mary said that he was so kind, had even complimented her by saying something along the lines that she was a good dancer. But as they bid adieu, he addressed her as lieutenant, adding that next time she wanted to pretend to be French she should remember to take off her GI watch.

She returned to her friends huddled together. They'd been watching her dance with General Bradley. One of the male officers who'd served with her since Fort Leonard Wood days was forever ribbing her and quipped, "Well, my fellow officers, leave it to Balster when there's rank in the room."

I caught a dim gleam in her eyes when she told me that story. It was her 90th birthday. For a few years she'd talked openly with me about her anxiety over the knowledge that she was experiencing short-term memory loss. She had been the director of a nursing home in the latter stages of her nursing career, so she knew the clinical stages of dementia. Before her war memories faded too, she wanted me to read the letters and interview her.

Mary had been 42 when I was born, so I had known only a few of the timeless heroes who lived in those letters. I met Lorraine when I was 16 at her home in Tacoma, Washington. At that point in my life, I wasn't even mildly curious about World War II, yet Lorraine insisted on telling me all about Mary when they were young. Certainly, I would never have guessed that I would call on the memories of Lorraine's stories several decades later and include them in a manuscript.

Some readers may think that I characterized Mary too critically, i.e., her persistent disregard for rules, the continual temptation to be impulsive, the half-truths she told herself to justify bad decisions. I fully admit to this characterization, but I hope that I also showed the genuine Mary, the young woman who, when push came to shove, found her instinctively heroic nature took over, and she became a practically minded, fully capable, incredibly loving, selfless caregiver—and above all, the most loving mother a child could ever hope for.

As many of the letters attest, it occurred to me that Inga's description of Mary having been "dumb like a fox" was accurate. But by the time I was done reading the archives and interviewing her, I concluded that Mary was dumb like a fox because she had to be.

When she was in her early nineties, she lived with me for two years. Her last memories were of the war, long after she'd forgotten the names of her children. One day during those two years she said that it was such a strange thing but that every time she woke from a nap or a good night's sleep the first thing that popped in her mind was a "long number." I asked her if she could tell me what the number was. She said yes. It was N-775-512. By then, I knew that it was her serial number, but I didn't tell her. Instead,

I asked her if she had any idea what the number referred to. She said she didn't have a clue.

Her last fears were of being too cold and of not being able to warm up. Her neurotic tendencies stayed with her too, as evidenced by my finding wads of Kleenex tissues underneath her pillow when I would make her bed. We children often teased her that she should have bought stock in Kleenex since she was obsessed with the product and would go into a "Mary maelstrom" if she couldn't find an unused one in her pocket.

One afternoon I woke her from napping because it was time for supper. She never liked the term "supper," said it was one of those "southern sayings." She preferred to call the evening meal "dinner." Anyway, after dozing heavily, she told me that she'd been having a nightmare about Chiefee. In the dream she was in deep trouble with Maxson because she was late reporting for duty. This prompted me to ask her if she dreamed about the war a lot. She didn't really know, she said, but she sure was hoping that she didn't dream about that mean woman anymore.

There are two specific anecdotes that Mary repeated to me that never ventured from the original stories, although both I find perplexing to this day because I never found enough satisfactory evidence to support either. The barn event was told to me when I was a little girl, but back then all she said was that two male officers along with two female officers were killed. She said that they had gone AWOL with two male officers who believed that a day excursion they planned would be safe. She said all four were killed. If it happened to these two "other nurses" and the two officers who'd accompanied them, all of whom did not survive, then how could Mary have known the specifics of the event when I pressed her to talk more about it when I was formally interviewing her for this project? Based on those interviews, all I can surmise is that either the event happened to her, Mona, and their beaus, or she dreamed that it did. I will attest that during her two-year stint with me, her dreams were so vivid and often she felt like talking about the most horrific memories just after she woke from her naps. Did her dreams unlock the real truth of the barn event, that it happened to her, Mona, W, and Bryson, not four people she barely knew?

There was another event that I never could reconcile as to whether it was something that happened to her or perhaps a mix of a dream with a true experience. I was tucking her in and putting in her eye drops that she always asked for right before she went to sleep. She asked me if I believed in God, and I said, "You know I have issues with all that, so why are you asking me?"

She replied, "Because you should believe. I know God is real, and I know that God answers prayers."

I asked her if she was going to repeat her mantra that "there are no atheists in foxholes." She said, "No, I'm going to tell you about the time that I was in a cellar for several days, and I prayed and prayed and three days later I was the only one who lived through that ordeal." I couldn't find any evidence in the letters about the cellar. But at that time, I didn't know there were two red volumes of letters. My oldest sister Madge was in possession of that other volume. A few years later, when I was still researching, Madge visited me and brought me that second volume. Many of the letters were the same as those in the volume I had been working from, but some of the letters contained in the second book were different. In the volume that Madge brought me, I found a November 30, 1944, letter that substantiated Mary's cellar experience:

> ... Our hospital was shelled two nites in succession. Still don't know if they didn't know we were a hospital, missed their target or just didn't care. Am referring to our enemy. Anyway, it was a horrible experience. Spent 3 nites in a cold dark, stinky cellar... When we came there wasn't a single pane of glass in any window, no heat and we wade thru mud holes out to the pump to get water, then carry it up 3 flights of stairs to our room. Now have little coal stoves in our rooms, but ours caught the floor on fire and the engineers had to knock out half the floor to get it out. The roof still leaks pretty badly, but these are all minor things compared to being afraid and then when we see what our poor boys endure up front...

In her service diary she chronicled the time in the cellar, this time stating that everyone survived. Had Mary dreamed that she was in a cellar for three days and was the only one to survive? Or did this really happen? I have no way of knowing. I did promise her that night that I would take God into consideration. She said, "Well, good. Now give me a kiss goodnight." I did, and this was the last time that she mentioned the cellar event to me.

The same day that she gave me the red volume containing the letters, she also handed me her service diary. After rifling through it for a few seconds, I asked her what happened to the last section, as it was clear that it had been torn out. She responded with a cryptic remark: "Oh, who knows why we do what we do when we're young." Her answer told me that I shouldn't pry, as it was obvious to me that she didn't care to tell me the entire truth. It was only after having read the letters and the diary that I understood. The last entry was about Robby coming to visit her in May 1945. She'd torn out the pages belonging to the summer of '45, the summer she spent with W.

Mary's sister Nancy told me over a phone call a few years ago that just after the war Mary returned home to "1262" and spent almost three months basically holed up in her childhood room. She hardly ever came out, ate very little, and talked even less. The shell of Mary returned, but it would take years for her to regain a fraction of the beguiling nature that defined her when she signed up for the army behind her parents' backs. Her three-month retreat to her St. Paul bedroom was her attempt to soothe a wrecked emotional state and try to find the young woman who used to live there. But that young woman hadn't survived the war.

Back then the service assigned the term "combat exhaustion" to describe post-war soldiers who suffered from emotional distress. But Mary wouldn't have been diagnosed as having it since, in the army's culture at the time, she couldn't possibly have suffered from combat exhaustion because she wasn't considered to be a post-war combat soldier.

She served on the front lines, yes. She took care of the mortally wounded. Yes. She was shot at. Yes. She got herself pinned up in a field with land mines. Yes. She suffered several concussions. Yes. She came very close to death from severe dehydration and hypothermia. Yes. She hit the ditch more times than she cared to count to take cover from Luftwaffe strafing. Yes. She came under siege with enemy combatants. Yes. She lived on the ground and was holed up a few miles from Bastogne when the Allies were surrounded by the enemy. Yes.

Yet neither she nor any of the female clinicians who served on the front lines of that war were considered to have been combat soldiers. Therefore, they couldn't have been diagnosed with "combat exhaustion." Today, of course, she would have been diagnosed with PTSD. I've now come to theorize that her three-month self-imposed imprisonment in the winter of 1945 was her way of attempting to come to terms with the PTSD that she didn't know she had.

During that time in her bedroom, I imagine that she was despondent but forced herself to try to say a mental goodbye to everyone she loved so dearly, especially those with whom she spent the war. When I think of all the people who meant so much to her, defined her, helped her figure out who she was—Zim, Redmond, W, Mona, Alabama, Poncho, all those boys and men with whom she'd held hands as they slipped away, pretending to be their mother when they called out "Mom" with uneven breaths—God, such loss. There must have been so many memories, heavy and complex.

Years later when Peter Riva was talking with me about Mary's love life, he asserted what I now believe is brilliantly accurate—the Mary who arrived at Fort Leonard Wood on March 31, 1943, did not return to St. Paul in November 1945. She didn't come back from that war. And that's what her father knew would happen. That's the reason he "threw a conniption."

Peter added that it was clear to him that Mary had to say goodbye to W because she'd shared that awful time with him and couldn't possibly have survived the emotional distress of daily living after the war if she'd chosen to live with a man who would remind her of it every day. Yes, Robby had also been in the war, but save for the times they shared on the *Andes*, the few visits with each other in Europe, or the couple of hours he saw her on December 10, 1944, he hadn't experienced the same war as she had with W. During the many years that I was trying to figure out how to write this manuscript, Peter's "read" was that I wasn't writing a war story, I was writing a love story. His assertion led to me to this—Mary's love for W couldn't exist outside of that horrific world they shared from spring of 1944 until August of 1945. Love like that doesn't belong outside of war. In a sense, maybe I did chronicle a war story by writing about a love that happened *because* of war and by writing about why that love ended for the same reason, *because* of war.

I know that many will want to know what happened after the war to Lorraine, Mona, Alabama, Redmond, and Poncho, but I only know about Lorraine. I met her on a trip to Tacoma, Washington, when I was 16 years old. She couldn't wait to meet me. She married a Navy guy named Pat, although I don't recall their last name. I recall that Lorraine made Baked Alaska while my sister Madge, her husband Jay, my mom, and I were visiting her. She was determined to tell me all about my mother and their antics growing up and their days at Fort Wood and in Tennessee. But Lorraine was removed from Tennessee maneuvers. I'm guessing that Mary was able to remain in touch with Lorraine because she didn't spend the actual war with her.

As far as the others, as beloved as they were, Mary did not remain in contact with them; therefore, I have no information on what happened to any of them. The trauma that my mother underwent during that war was so terrible that she never overcame it. I'm now certain that the reason she didn't keep up with Mona, with Alabama, with so many of the people she shared the war with was because she couldn't. She had to hold them inside a place in her head where she could keep them in that time. It had to be a separate and distinct time that had nothing to do with her future life. She didn't keep up with them because she couldn't emotionally incorporate them into a life back in the States post war. They didn't belong there.

Only recently I've begun to formulate a theory as to why she didn't, couldn't involve them in her life after the war. I think it's because my mother died during that war, not physically, but she died all the same. And the people who were with her died, too. She viewed the life that she took up post war as a re-birth, and notwithstanding the innocent stories she told me about Mona, Alabama, and others, she couldn't bring them with her to her post-war world. She kept them in some sort of time capsule that I forced her to open during the interviews more than 70 years later.

My mother was smart. She must have known that she was taking a big emotional risk to allow me to interview her. But her need to honor those people she loved so much during that time in her life overruled her lifelong habit to repress all that pain.

Maybe I've spent the last 12 years of my life writing this manuscript as a way of sorting through the emotional contradictions that Mary could never reconcile. I've finally quit worrying about whether anyone ever reads this story. The reason I wrote the story was to help my mother find closure, although I'm sure that I failed to do that. I've bet myself many times that she was dreaming about the war when she drew her last breath during the Covid-19 pandemic when she was six months shy of her 100th birthday.

I do think that Robby and Mary were madly in love after having known each other only ten days on the *Andes*, so at the time, it made complete sense that they would promise to marry. Maybe they shared some sort of magical thinking that if they planned to get married after the war then such a decision would force fate to guarantee they'd both survive it. But this is not to say that they didn't love each other. On the contrary. I'll assume that my siblings witnessed their love for each other just as I did every day of childhood.

She used to say to me, "Your daddy wasn't in as much danger during the war as I was." What she really meant by that was that Robby had more capacity to put the war in its place, in the past, than she was able to. He lived in the present, and the only time that the war showed up for him was post-surgery in heavy dream states while anesthesia was wearing off. He'd yell, "Get the rope. Get the God-damned rope," which may have been associated with some artillery reference. I can't be sure because, even after two written requests to the U.S. Army in which I included a copy of his death certificate and his serial number, they've never sent me his service records.

My father used to entertain all of us kids with his great gift for storytelling. But there was only one repeated anecdote that had a war association that I remember. He and Mary had been married about a year and already had Madge, the first of their six kids. The story goes that they were living in El Paso and Mary answered the phone one evening during dinnertime. Apparently, Robby overheard Mary saying to the person on the line that no, he couldn't possibly fly down to El Paso, that she was married and had a little baby, at which point Robby took the phone from her and said to the caller that he'd killed hundreds of Germans during the war and wouldn't hesitate to add another bastard to his list of kills. Then he said that he hung up the phone and that they never heard from the "sonuvabitch" again. It wasn't until five or six years after my father died that I read Mary's letters and service diary and put together that the phone call had most likely been from W.

NCR Davis